E____ Right from 8 to 18

Eating Right from 8 to 18

Nutrition Solutions for Parents

Sandra K. Nissenberg, M.S., R.D.
and Barbara N. Pearl, M.S., R.D.

John Wiley & Sons, Inc.

Published by John Wiley & Sons, Inc., New York
Published simultaneously in Canada

This publication is designed to provide accurate and authoritative information in
regard to the subject matter covered. It is sold with the understanding that the
publisher is not engaged in rendering professional services. If professional advice or
other expert assistance is required, the services of a competent professional person
should be sought.

Library of Congress Cataloging-in-Publication Data:

Nissenberg, Sandra K.
    Eating right from 8 to 18 : nutrition solutions for parents / Sandra K.
Nissenberg and Barbara N. Pearl.
        p. cm.
        Includes index.
        ISBN 0-471-39282-0 (pbk.)
        1. Eating disorders in children. 2. Obesity in children—Prevention. 3.
Children—Nutrition—Psychological aspects. I. Title: Eating right from
eight to eighteen. II. Pearl, Barbara N. III. Title.

RJ506.E18 N57 2002
613.2′083—dc21   2001046862

Printed in the United States of America
10 9 8 7 6 5 4 3 2 1

CONTENTS

INTRODUCTION

You are what you eat! How many times in your life have you heard this phrase? But have you ever really *thought* about it?

When we were young, we constantly heard our parents say things like: "Eat your vegetables"; "No snacks, it's too close to dinnertime"; "Drink your milk, it's good for you." Most times we *reluctantly* did as we were told, but we couldn't really understand why. And, of course, we believed that when we became parents ourselves, we wouldn't make our kids eat things we didn't ourselves like to eat. We would be different. But now . . . have we become our parents?

Sometime about the time we became parents ourselves, we began to realize just how important nutrition and the foods we eat really are. Our unconditional love for our children makes us want them to be the healthiest, strongest, and happiest they can be. And as parents we can help build them into healthy, happy adults by nurturing and nourishing them properly. Sometimes we think we know what's right (because we're *parents,* after all) and other times we go by what we hear from others, read in the popular press, or see on TV.

But it is so difficult to keep up with all of the latest research and make sure that we're really telling and giving our children what is best for them. Plus, as our children grow, often we find that their individual quirks make it difficult to give them a nutritionally sound foundation. So, in this book, we are going to present the most current information on foods; what should be eaten; how we can raise our children to make wise choices about the foods they eat; and how to handle various nutrition-related concerns that might arise over the years between eight and eighteen, as these years are so crucial in establishing lifelong habits and are vital growth years. We share knowledgeable information, answer common questions, and offer direction on what's a parent to do.

Part One of the book opens with information that allows you to assess the nutritional status of your child. The information provided on proper growth and development, dietary guidelines, and nutrient requirements for various age groups will assist you in determining how well your child is meeting his or her particular nutrition needs.

Part Two proceeds with solutions for managing various nutrition-related concerns. Weight loss or gain, eating disorders, vegetarianism, picky eaters, special needs for competitive athletes, and food allergies and intolerances are just some of the concerns addressed. We'll show you what to do if you suspect one of these concerns is applicable to your child, and help lay the groundwork for making sure your child starts to realize that nutrition has a strong connection to living a happy, healthy life.

Part Three is filled with practical, specific directions to implement all your "food smarts" so that you can become a good role model yourself; shop knowledgeably in the grocery store; learn how to fix a healthy brown-bag lunch for your child; and still eat smart when you eat out and have a snack. The final section of the book offers you a collection of over a hundred healthy recipes that will instill balance, variety, and good nutrition into your family's diet. And at the very end is a list of support groups, resource organizations, and Web sites.

As registered dietitians with more than forty years combined experience, and as parents ourselves, we know what's healthy and how to get kids to eat right. We also know the common struggles parents go through on a daily basis. In this book, we do our best to take scientific knowledge and bring it to you in practical, easy-to-understand *nutrition solutions for parents.*

All in all, from the information contained within these pages, you should be able to educate your children from an early age about the benefits of good nutrition (and learn something that will help your own nutritional status too!). You'll now have the answers you need to tackle a wide range of nutrition concerns and be able to pass adequate information on to your children which, in turn, can be of benefit to many more generations to come.

We wish you happy, healthy eating for you and your family.

PART ONE

ASSESSING YOUR CHILD'S NUTRITION STATUS

1

IS MY CHILD HEALTHY?
Looking at Your Child's Eating Habits and Weight

How many times have you questioned the eating habits of your child? It's second nature for a parent to worry—worry about how much milk Johnny drinks, or how many daily snacks Melanie eats, or even how often David eats fast food each week.

What makes children poor eaters? What makes children healthy eaters? What makes them gain or lose weight? We'll get into that, but let's first try to assess your overall nutrition knowledge and your child's nutritional status. With this information you can determine what specific nutrition concerns you need to concentrate on and establish a course of action.

To start, let's check your basic nutrition IQ.

Nutrition IQ: What Do You Know?

1. Your mom always told you to drink your milk. How much milk should your teenager be drinking each day?
   a. one serving
   b. two servings
   c. three or more servings

2. You know that calcium is important. Which of these foods supply calcium in the diet?
   a. milk
   b. yogurt
   c. green, leafy vegetables

    d. sardines

    e. all of the above

3. It's time for an afternoon snack. Which is your best choice?
    a. potato chips
    b. frozen yogurt cone
    c. candy bar
    d. sunflower seeds

4. Your child is involved in outdoor sports. It's hot and dry outside. Which is the best beverage to keep on hand?
    a. soft drink
    b. sweetened sports drink
    c. water

5. Fiber is important in the diet. Which of the following foods best contribute fiber?
    a. carrot sticks
    b. apple
    c. whole wheat crackers
    d. raisin bran cereal
    e. all of the above

6. You want to keep extra pounds from creeping on. What's the best plan of action?
    a. seek the latest quick weight loss plan
    b. eat healthy foods
    c. skip meals
    d. remove all fat from your diet

7. One day your ten-year-old daughter declares her intention to become a vegetarian. What snack food would contribute the greatest amount of protein?
    a. string cheese
    b. apple
    c. vanilla wafers
    d. popcorn

8. You're running to soccer practice and there's no time to make dinner. Fast food appears to be the only option tonight. What's the most nutritious choice?
    a. taco salad
    b. hamburger

   c. tuna salad sub sandwich

   d. pepperoni personal pan pizza

Answers:

1. c. Teens require as much as 1,300 mg. of calcium/day, and that can be obtained in 3 to 4 servings of milk.
2. e. All of these foods would contribute calcium to the diet.
3. b. A frozen yogurt cone is your healthiest choice, being lowest in fat. Potato chips, candy, and even sunflower seeds supply more fat and less nutrition.
4. c. Water is the best choice to rehydrate the body and replace fluids lost through sweating.
5. e. All of these foods contribute fiber to the diet and are wise choices.
6. b. Eating healthy food choices can help you maintain and even lose weight in the long run without feeling deprived of food. Fad dieting, skipping meals, and eliminating fat can all lead to additional food and nutrition problems.
7. a. Although any of those listed would be good snack options, string cheese supplies the greatest amount of protein at 7.0 grams/stick.
8. b. A hamburger with lettuce, tomatoes, onions, or any other vegetable would be the best option, supplying the least amount of fat and calories. A single hamburger weighs in at 260 calories and 9 grams of fat, while each of the other options supplies between 500 and 900 calories and 28 to 52 grams of fat.

How well did you do? Nutrition is so important it should be a big part of our lives and those of our children. Good health is a prized possession. It cannot be bought, only acquired from good habits. But good habits are *years* in the making. Many times a person's health is taken for granted until a diagnosis to the contrary occurs. When this happens, it then becomes necessary to stop, take notice, and do what it takes to gain a healthy status again. But by then it may be too late. Children are rarely concerned with their future health; it's something they take for granted. They just assume that they will feel good forever, and live to a ripe old age. But as parents, we know otherwise. That's why we, as parents, need to give guidance to our children and set examples by establishing and maintaining a healthy lifestyle.

Fortunately, times have never presented us with better opportunities for obtaining good health. We know more now than ever before about what promotes good health and what contributes to health problems. We can use this knowledge to make choices to promote our own and our children's overall health and wellbeing, and delay and even prevent the onset of disease. This information is available to anyone who chooses to seek it, and we would be foolish to overlook what is so widely available to us.

We also know that people develop food habits early in life. Habits formed before the age of six are likely to continue through the years and have the maximum effect on overall health and quality of life. Parents, peers, and environmental surroundings all contribute to these eating patterns and behaviors, so you should start focusing right now on improving your child's eating habits and food choices.

FOODNOTE
Healthy habits established early in life are the foundation of good health throughout life.

Is My Child Eating Healthy?

Here we want you to analyze how you and your child are doing in terms of your eating habits each day.

How Well Do You Eat? How Well Does Your Child Eat?

Choose an answer from each of the following groupings that best pertains to you; then the answer that pertains to your child.

a. I (my child) eat/eats as much as 6 to 11 servings of whole grain breads, cereals, crackers, rice, or pasta daily.
b. I (my child) choose/chooses whole grain products at least 3 to 5 times per week.
c. I (my child) prefer/prefers white bread over whole wheat and typically eats 1 to 3 servings daily.

a. I (my child) eat/eats 3 or more vegetables daily.
b. I (my child) eat/eats 1 or 2 vegetables daily.
c. I (my child) choose/chooses a salad occasionally with dinner.

a. I (my child) eat/eats 2 or 3 fruits daily.
b. I (my child) eat/eats 1 fruit each day.

   c. Occasionally, I (my child) snack/snacks on a banana or some grapes, but rarely eat/eats fruit otherwise.

   a. I (my child) eat/eats lean meat, poultry, fish, dried beans or tofu 2 or 3 times daily.

   b. I (my child) choose/chooses lean meat products 1 or 2 times weekly.

   c. I (my child) prefer/prefers hamburgers, fried chicken, or steak over lean meat products.

   a. I (my child) eat/eats 2 or 3 servings of low-fat dairy products (milk, yogurt, cheese) daily.

   b. I (my child) sometimes choose/chooses low-fat dairy products and sometimes whole milk and ice cream.

   c. I (my child) would choose whole milk and regular ice cream over low-fat milk and frozen yogurt.

   a. I (my child) exercise/exercises at least 3 times weekly for at least 30 minutes each time.

   b. I (my child) exercise/exercises once or twice a week for 20 to 30 minutes.

   c. I (my child) occasionally walk/walks for exercise.

Number of "a" answers
Myself _____ × 3 = _____   My Child _____ × 3 = _____
Number of "b" answers
Myself _____ × 2 = _____   My Child _____ × 2 = _____
Number of "c" answers
Myself _____ × 1 = _____   My Child _____ × 1 = _____

Now add up the points for yourself, and then for your child.

If you (or your child) scored . . .

Total of 15 to 18 points, you (or your child) are doing great with your eating and exercise habits. Keep up the good work.

Total of 11 to 14 points, you (or your child) could use a little improvement. You need to add more variety into your choices, watch fat intake, and increase regular exercise habits.

Total of 10 or less points, you (or your child) need some help and guidance. By following the suggestions and guidance found in this book, you can begin to move in the right direction. Good luck!!

We all can benefit from learning all we can about nutrition and its effect on health. The science of nutrition is constantly changing, and children go through so many changes . . . all of which are a part of growing up.

These enormous transitions all tie in with lifestyle habits, and nutrition is a big part of this picture. Babies grow at a tremendous rate, doubling their weight in five months and tripling it in a year. Although they grow at a somewhat slower pace, our toddlers, preschoolers, and school-aged kids continue to grow rapidly in front of our eyes. But somewhere between the ages of fifteen and eighteen children enter their final major growth spurt. Here Mother Nature helps them grow into their adult bodies. For boys, adding extra muscle and increased blood volume is standard. For girls, collecting some extra fat padding (most likely in undesirable places) is likely. Sometimes these changes are not what our children have in mind for their own shapes and bodies, so they try to force Mother Nature's plans on a different course. Boys often overeat to bulk up, while girls may choose to undereat in order to stay slim. Neither is a good choice and both can lead to health problems in later years. Eating right and making wise food choices are important to properly feeding and fueling the body. To do so, a good, positive attitude about food is a must, along with eating a variety of foods that build and nourish the body properly.

As children grow and seek greater independence, they sometimes use food as a bargaining or negotiating tool. Food and healthy eating often become control issues. This is often the case with eating disorders, vegetarianism, and overweight conditions. Teens and young adults not only receive conflicting messages about foods they eat and don't eat (some good and others not so good), they know that their parents are affected by their food intake. It's especially easy for young people to grow up with unhealthy feelings about foods as they receive so many mixed messages about how much they should weigh, how they should look, and where they can get the perfect body.

FOODNOTE

Good eating habits are *just as easy* to create as bad ones are!

Our responsibility as parents lies in what we *offer* our children to eat and what we make available to them. Ultimately, it's our children's responsibility to eat or not to eat; we can't force foods on them.

Reasons to Eat Healthy

- Eating healthy shows you care about your body and your health
- Eating healthy makes you feel good, giving you energy to work, play, and feel your best

- Eating healthy gives you the opportunity to think more clearly for yourself
- Eating healthy helps your immediate family, extended family, and future generations learn to eat right as well
- Eating healthy builds good attitudes about foods and reduces the likelihood of future eating problems
- Eating healthy gives you a positive outlook on life
- Eating healthy sets the foundation for a lifetime of health and reduction of disease

As children move from childhood to adulthood, they encounter many changes. Sometimes their bodies grow so fast they are not quite comfortable with their physical and emotional selves. It takes several years to understand all of the changes. Growth spurts, acne problems, hormone changes, menstruation in girls, and putting up a fight for independence are just some of the more common events preteens and teenagers go through. It is important to reassure your child that these changes are normal—and you can start by knowing, and informing, your children about what's a healthy weight for them.

What's a Healthy Weight for My Child?

A weight chart alone cannot determine a healthy weight. So many of us have had the unpleasant experience of being weighed, or watching our child being weighed, at the doctor's office and being told we, or our child, weigh too much for our height, according to the chart on the wall. This method is outdated. The chart does not take into account muscle weight versus fat weight.

There is a difference between being muscular, being overweight, and being obese. Obesity indicates that a person has excess body fat. Being overweight could mean a person is obese, but it could also indicate that one has a large muscle mass. Most athletes are overweight because of their muscles, not because they have too much body fat. This can also be true for active teen athletes. Thus the weight charts would not be appropriate indication of healthy weight for these teens.

When children visit their doctor, heights and weights are charted on graphs developed by the National Center for Health Statistics in collaboration with the Centers for Disease Control and Prevention. Most pediatricians will provide these charts in the child's medical records so they can be referenced through the growing years.

The charts on pages 10–11 illustrate the normal range of height and weight for American boys and girls up to eighteen years of age. Children's heights and weights are shown in percentiles. For example, a child of average height for a particular age would be in the fiftieth percentile; a tall child in the ninety-fifth percentile; a short child in the fifth percentile. Weight is treated in a similar manner. After plotting height and weight on these charts over a period of years, patterns emerge that show how your child may or may not be growing properly. But remember, these are just *guides* to follow—they don't tell the whole story.

After all, every child grows differently. One teenage boy may be the smallest in the class until he hits his fourteenth birthday; then he may shoot up to be the tallest. A young girl may hit her maximum growth by the time she reaches fifteen. Thus the preteen and teen years are important periods of growth and development. Nutritional requirements during this time frame are extremely important for building tissues, muscles, bones, blood volume, and much more.

As of June 1998, nutrition experts have devised another method to determine height and weight status of Americans. The National Heart, Lung and Blood Institute developed these guidelines in cooperation with the National Institute of Diabetes and Digestive and Kidney Diseases. Referred to as Body Mass Index or BMI, this easy-to-use method is based on gender, current weight, and height, and provides information on whether a person is at a healthy weight or is underweight or overweight. The charts, on pages 12–13, are different for boys and for girls. Please note the formula provided on the charts (in the upper left) so that you can calculate your child's BMI.

The following indicates whether your child is at a healthy weight or not:

Healthy weight = BMI of 19–24.9

Overweight = BMI of 25–29.9

Obese = BMI of 30 or more

In terms of percentiles:

Underweight	BMI-for-age ≤ 5th percentile
At risk of overweight	BMI-for-age ≥ 85th percentile
Overweight	BMI-for-age ≥ 95th percentile

(continued on page 14)

Growth Chart for Boys

2 to 20 Years: Boys' Stature and Weight for Age

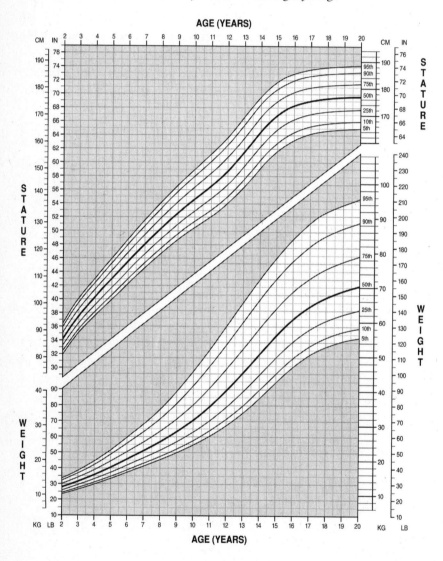

Growth Chart for Girls

2 to 20 Years: Girls' Stature and Weight for Age

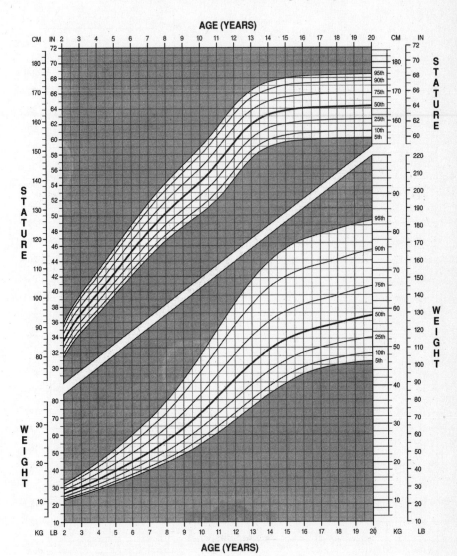

Body Mass Index Chart for Boys

2 to 20 Years: Boys' Body Mass Index-for-Age Percentiles

NAME _____

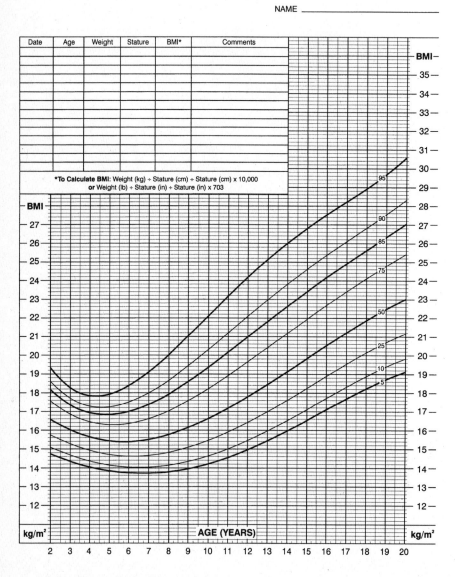

Date	Age	Weight	Stature	BMI*	Comments

*To Calculate BMI: Weight (kg) ÷ Stature (cm) ÷ Stature (cm) x 10,000
or Weight (lb) ÷ Stature (in) ÷ Stature (in) x 703

AGE (YEARS)

SOURCE: Developed by the National Center for Health Statistics in collaboration with
the National Center for Chronic Disease Prevention and Health Promotion (2000).
http://www.cdc.gov/growthcharts

Body Mass Index Chart for Girls

2 to 20 Years: Girls' Body Mass Index-for-Age Percentiles

NAME _____

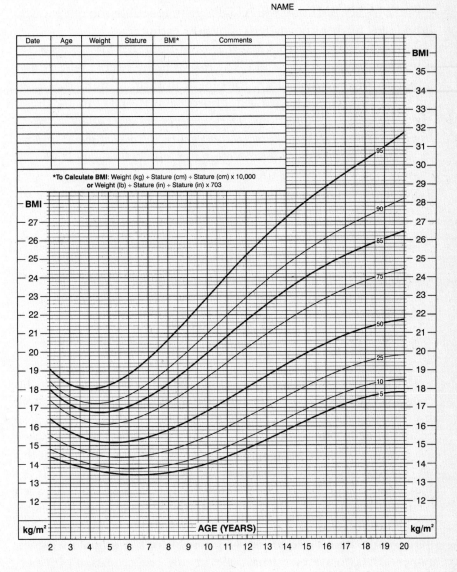

Date	Age	Weight	Stature	BMI*	Comments

*To Calculate BMI: Weight (kg) ÷ Stature (cm) ÷ Stature (cm) x 10,000
or Weight (lb) ÷ Stature (in) ÷ Stature (in) x 703

BMI

35
34
33
32
31
30
29
28
27
26
25
24
23
22
21
20
19
18
17
16
15
14
13
12

kg/m²

AGE (YEARS)

2 3 4 5 6 7 8 9 10 11 12 13 14 15 16 17 18 19 20

SOURCE: Developed by the National Center for Health Statistics in collaboration with
the National Center for Chronic Disease Prevention and Health Promotion (2000).
http://www.cdc.gov/growthcharts

13

(continued)

These standards are generous, yet the rate of obesity in our children has risen drastically from 5 percent in 1964 to almost 13 percent in 1994, with further increases into the new millennium.

Now look at the table to determine where your child's weight falls. If your child's weight falls into the normal range or slightly above normal, you do not need to be overly concerned. But, if you see a trend toward a higher BMI or if your child is gaining weight too quickly, you should seek further knowledge on healthy eating.

However, some doctors feel that even though BMI is important in helping determine if a child is at risk of being overweight, it may be better for parents to look for practical warning signs that their child may or may not have a weight problem. Parents can ask themselves the following questions: *Does my child get short of breath easily during exercise? Does my child's weight get in the way of social or physical events? Does my child wear clothing to hide her weight?* If you, as a parent, answer "yes" to these types of questions, you need to seek guidance on dealing with these weight-related issues and you'll want to concentrate on Part Two of this book.

FOODNOTE

Studies show the earlier one starts dieting (childhood vs. adolescence vs. adulthood), the higher one's weight becomes in adulthood.

Determining if a young person is underweight is often more difficult. Visual assessment by a parent or close friend sometimes helps in spotting an underweight child. Generally, a growth chart in the child's medical record can be helpful. If the child's weight seems to have taken a drastic dive downward at any point, and his or her height stops increasing, this can be a sign of excessive weight loss and possible slowed growth. If the chart shows a large difference (as determined by the physician) between weight and height, this can be a sign of disproportionate weight for height.

The possibility of an eating disorder needs to be considered when there is an extreme weight loss (25 percent of the original weight), ammenorrhea (loss of menstrual cycle) in girls, preoccupation with dieting, fear of becoming fat, no known illness leading to weight loss, and/or refusal to maintain a normal weight. Many times, eating disorders are tied into a person's body image.

Body image is the way someone views how his or her body looks. It also includes what people believe others think about their appearance. Often, body image reflects people's general feelings about themselves. Sometimes, it's easier to focus on weight than on more serious problems. It's more acceptable in our society to say, "I feel fat" than "I'm depressed."

FOODNOTE

Too many kids base their looks and body size on their primary sense of self-worth.

Most girls and boys between the ages of eight to eighteen years are very concerned with the physical changes that occur to them. Adolescence is a time of rapid growth and physical change. Teens have not grown this fast since infancy and will not grow this rapidly again the rest of their lives. In addition, teens go through puberty, which can last anywhere from two to six years. Puberty brings hormones, which bring many bodily changes. Some of these changes can be uncomfortable and may take time to get used to. Yet teens want to be just the right height and weight, have the right look, and develop "normally" sexually. They don't want to stand out in a crowd. Teens often feel that being fat or thin will determine how smart they are, if they'll have friends, and even if they'll be successful in life.

Girls, in particular, spend a great deal of their adolescence reading teen and fashion magazines and comparing themselves to models and TV stars. Through these media, they learn about the newest diet trend, diet aid, diet pill, and techniques such as vomiting and laxative use to keep the weight off. Unfortunately, being thin and attractive becomes a greater priority than their health.

FOODNOTE

About 10 percent of eating disorders start before the age of 10; 33 percent between the ages of eleven and fifteen; and more than 50 percent between the ages of sixteen and twenty.

Young people are even starting to worry about their weight earlier and earlier. Studies have shown that by fourth and fifth grades as many as 80 percent of the girls have already been on a diet to lose weight. But girls do not own this world of body image problems. Boys, too, are self-conscious about how they look. Where girls may want to be pencil thin, boys want to be muscular and buff.

FOODNOTE

If the measurements of a Barbie doll were projected to a life-size woman, she would have a 36-inch bust, 18-inch waist, and 33-inch hips. A life-size G. I. Joe would have 27-inch biceps. In other words, models of unrealistic body images are being presented to our children.

Constant reassurance needs to be given to our kids to emphasize that they are "OK" and that the differences they see between themselves and their friends are normal. Their feelings regarding their fatness or thinness are often unrealistic. It's important to encourage your child not to go on a weight loss diet, but instead to learn how to eat healthier. You'll find out how in the following pages.

2

STARTING YOUNG
Making Sure Your Child Is Getting the Basics Right Now

One of the hardest things for today's parents is how to know if their children are eating a balanced diet. One reason is that nutrition advice seems to be changing all the time. So many people are willing to offer conflicting opinions—and this includes the media, relatives, employees of health food stores, researchers, and friends. But often the information given is confusing and misleading. We are here to give you a good foundation of sound nutrition information that will help you determine whether your child is meeting the basics of a healthy diet.

Back in the 1950s the United States Department of Agriculture created the Basic 4 Food Groups (meat, dairy, fruits/vegetables, and breads/cereals) and recommended amounts to be eaten from each group. Today, this plan has been modified to the Food Guide Pyramid, which emphasizes balance and moderation by illustrating how to build a healthy diet by eating more from one group and less from another. By following this guide you can be assured that you and your family will be eating healthy. This pyramid places more emphasis on nutrient-rich foods and less emphasis on those foods that are higher in sugar and fat. So should you and your child.

From the bottom up (the groups we are supposed to eat the most of are at the bottom of the pyramid), the groups are:

1. breads, starches, cereal, rice, pasta
2. vegetables
3. fruits

Food Guide Pyramid
A Guide to Daily Food Choices

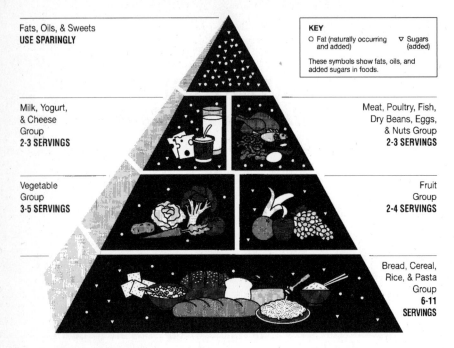

The Food Guide Pyramid

4. milk, dairy products, yogurt, cheese
5. meat, poultry, fish, eggs, dried beans
6. fats, oils, sugars, sweets

FOODNOTE

Remember three words: balance, variety, moderation.

The pyramid helps us with balancing our food choices; in selecting a variety of foods; and with eating in moderation. How do we realistically do this on a daily basis?

• *Balancing Food Choices:* Choose foods from *different* groups during the *same* meal. Selecting a food from each of the food groups helps to plan well-balanced meals for you and your family.

• *Selecting a Variety of Foods:* Select a *variety* from within each group during the day. No one food can provide all the nutrients our body needs to stay healthy. By choosing a variety of foods each day, you will ensure yourself of the nutrients you need.

• *Eating in Moderation:* Eat portions that are adequate in size. All foods should be eaten in reasonable amounts. Even a healthy food can contribute to poor health if it is overeaten. Learn what portion sizes are appropriate—and we'll help you understand what they are.

Eating the Right Amount from the Food Groups Each Day

The number of servings we need to eat from each food group is dependent upon our gender, body size, and level of activity. The following calorie level guideline is based on recommendations of the National Academy of Sciences and on food consumption surveys.

CALORIE LEVEL GUIDELINES (PER DAY)

1,500–1,600 calories = the amount consumed by many sedentary women and older adults.

2,000–2,200 calories = the amount for most children, teenage girls, active women, and many sedentary men.

2,800 calories = the amount for teenage boys, many active men, and very active women.

Based on the food groups, here is a recommended daily serving plan for all three calorie levels:

Food Group (servings)	1,500–1,600 calories	2,000–2,200 calories	2,800 calories
breads, starches cereal, rice, pasta	6	9	11
vegetables	3	4	5
fruits	2	3	4
milk, dairy products, yogurt, cheese*	2–3	2–3	2–3
meat, poultry, fish, eggs, dried beans	5 oz.	6 oz.	7 oz.

*Teens require additional servings from this group to support growth and development.

Understanding Serving Sizes

The serving size listed on a product tells us how much a portion is—according to the manufacturer. This can be tricky, as the listed serving size could be larger than what is appropriate for some people to eat. But don't worry; you don't have to measure or weigh everything you eat. Over time, you'll learn to create an "eye" for appropriate portions by noting what seems right for you and your children. Also, keep in mind that some foods include servings from *more* than one group, so while the number of servings suggested may seem high, it's really not. Pizza, for example, includes foods from the starch, vegetable, dairy, and maybe even the meat groups. The same holds true with foods like hamburgers, cheeseburgers, tacos, casseroles, and soups.

To help you get a handle on serving size, here are some suggested serving sizes of commonly eaten foods:

Breads, Starches, Cereal, Rice, Pasta **(each serving size is about the size of *a woman's fist*):**

> 1 slice bread
>
> $\frac{1}{2}$ hamburger bun, hot dog bun, English muffin, or bagel
>
> 1 8-inch tortilla
>
> 5 or 6 crackers
>
> 1 small dinner roll
>
> 5 mini or 1 large rice cake
>
> 1 ounce ready-to-eat cereal or pretzels
>
> $\frac{1}{2}$ cup cooked cereal, rice, or pasta
>
> 12 tortilla chips
>
> 9 animal crackers

Vegetables **(a serving size is about the size of *a tennis ball*):**

> 1 cup raw, leafy vegetables
>
> $\frac{1}{2}$ cup cooked or nonleafy vegetables
>
> 7 or 8 baby carrots
>
> 2 spears broccoli
>
> 1 medium ear of corn
>
> 1 small potato
>
> 6 ounces vegetable juice
>
> 1 cup vegetable soup

Fruits **(a serving size is about the size of *a medium apple*):**

> 1 medium apple, banana, orange, or nectarine
>
> $\frac{1}{4}$ cantaloupe melon

$\frac{1}{8}$ honeydew melon

$\frac{1}{2}$ grapefruit

12 grapes

$\frac{1}{2}$ cup chopped, cooked, or canned fruit

$\frac{1}{4}$ cup dried fruit

6 ounces fruit juice

Milk, Dairy Products, Yogurt, Cheese:

1 cup milk or yogurt

1 cup frozen yogurt

$1\frac{1}{2}$ cups ice milk

$1\frac{1}{2}$ ounces natural cheese

2 ounces processed cheese

Meat, Poultry, Fish, Eggs, Dried Beans (a serving size of 3 ounces is about the size of *the palm of your hand or a deck of cards*):

2 to 3 ounces cooked lean meat, poultry, or fish

$\frac{1}{2}$ cup cooked dried beans

1 egg or 2 egg whites

2 tablespoons peanut butter

$\frac{1}{3}$ cup nuts

Your Child's Food Intake

You can track what your child eats on a daily basis by keeping a food chart or diary of what is eaten. You can also keep track of the number of servings from each food group. You may be surprised at the actual intake, and may need to increase or decrease the intake of certain food groups, based on the recommended portions of the food pyramid. Here's a sample chart.

MY CHILD'S DAILY INTAKE:

	bread/starch servings	vegetable servings	fruit servings	milk servings	meat servings	fat/ sweets
Breakfast	____	____	____	____	____	____
Lunch	____	____	____	____	____	____
Dinner	____	____	____	____	____	____
Snacks	____	____	____	____	____	____
Totals	____	____	____	____	____	____

Each time your child chooses a food, mark which food group it comes from. At the end of the day, tally up your totals to see how he/she rates.

Guidelines to Follow for Your Child's Daily Diet

The Dietary Guidelines for Americans were developed to serve as a standard for the United States population. Federal nutrition programs, like food stamps, school breakfast and lunch, and WIC (Women, Infants and Children Supplemental Nutrition) programs, are all impacted by these guidelines. (In fact, the Food Guide Pyramid is based on these guidelines!)

Intended for healthy children over age two and all healthy adults, the Dietary Guidelines help send messages about the importance of nutrition and fitness to overall health. To make these messages easy to remember and understand, the guidelines were revised in 2000 to emphasize three basic messages: A, B, and C.

- A = Aim for Fitness
  Aim for a healthy weight.
  Be physically active each day.

- B = Build a Healthy Base
  Let the Pyramid guide your food choices.
  Eat a variety of grains daily, especially whole grains.
  Eat a variety of fruits and vegetables daily.
  Keep foods safe to eat.

- C = Choose Sensibly
  Choose a diet that is low in saturated fat and
    cholesterol and moderate in total fat.
  Choose beverages and foods to moderate your intake
    of sugars.
  Choose and prepare foods with less salt.
  If you drink alcoholic beverages, do so in moderation.

Let's look at the ABCs in more detail.

A = Aim for Fitness

- *Aim for a healthy weight.* Being too heavy or too thin can lead to health problems. An ideal, healthy weight should be based on one's age, height, genetic background, body composition, body build, and physical activity level. It is very common for many pre-teens and teens to feel insecure about their body weight, but obsessing at a young age can lead to a lifetime preoccupation with weight. It is important for children to develop self-confidence and a positive self-image to help them feel good about their size. For example, tell your child, if she/he weighs too much, that not everyone can be tall, thin, and a size 6. Teach the value of eating healthfully over the idea of just being thin. And talk about the importance of healthy food to your children, emphasizing that food is a necessary component of life. These should be the first steps in helping to build this positive self-image in your children.

• *Be physically active each day.* It is well documented that moderate physical activity is important for good health. Physical activity is greatly related to improvements in flexibility and bone mass density, reduced incidence of depression and anxiety, reduction of disease, and maintenance of overall health in adults. In children, the benefits include greater muscular strength, aerobic endurance, and bone health. Being active can be as simple as walking briskly each day for twenty minutes, or kicking a soccer ball around with your youngster.

B = Build a Healthy Base

• *Let the Pyramid guide your food choices.* There are *many* healthy food choices. However, they all contribute different nutrients to the diet, so we need to vary our daily choices. Milk, for example, is an excellent source of calcium but contains no Vitamin C, something orange juice is packed with. So you may want your child to drink some orange juice at breakfast, but milk at lunch. Look back to the Food Guide Pyramid if you need clarification about recommended food groups and daily servings.

• *Eat a variety of grains daily, especially whole grains.* Once we believed that carbohydrates were making us too fat. Today there are still many popular weight loss diets that blame carbohydrates for weight gain. But this is not the case at all. Carbohydrates are the body's *best* source of energy. They are the easiest and quickest nutrients to digest, and are an accessible and abundant choice for many people, especially children and teens.

Carbohydrates are divided into two types: complex carbohydrates (starches and fibers) and sugars (simple carbohydrates). Complex carbohydrates are the carbohydrates of choice. Whole grain products and starchy vegetables like potatoes, dried beans, and peas are all rich in complex carbohydrates. These foods are also sources of fiber, important for digestion and elimination of bodily wastes. Generally, complex carbohydrates take longer to digest, thereby keeping us more satisfied with what we've eaten and less hungry overall. So serve your child that heaping spoonful of mashed potatoes, or offer a five-bean dip with some chips.

• *Eat a variety of fruits and vegetables daily.* Most people lack a plan for eating an adequate number of fruits and vegetables (often referred to as a 5 A Day plan). People of all ages should aim to include a *mini-mum* of five fruits and/or vegetables in their diet daily. This could trans-late into three fruits and two vegetables, or two fruits and three vegetables, or any other such combination. These foods contribute many healthy nutrients without excessive amounts of fat and sugar. They also add fiber, which helps to move food through the digestive system faster while making us feel full and satisfied. When your child asks for a snack, reach for an apple first. Offer candy and sweets as a last resort.

• *Keep foods safe to eat.* Food safety issues have *never* been so hot. It is a known fact that millions of people each year are affected by eat-ing contaminated foods. But most are cases of stomachaches, diarrhea, nausea, headaches, and vomiting—with only a small number being fatal. Yet these are the ones we hear about in the news, that scare us from eat-ing the food placed before us. Warnings about possible food contami-nation and foodborne illnesses often scare us into wondering if that apple picked off a tree is safe to eat, or if a hamburger at a fast food restaurant is cooked well enough, or even if food prepared in our own kitchens could have been contaminated on the countertop when we used one instead of two knives. *How can we be sure foods are safe?* What signs do we need to look for and be aware of in order to protect our families from harmful foods?

We need to eat—we know that. So what we need to understand is how we can best obtain and serve safe foods. The following is a chart of a few food safety precautions to keep in mind when preparing and handling food:

FOOD SAFETY GUIDE

1. Keep hands clean. Wash them again if you handled dirty dishes or the trash or used the bathroom. Make sure chil-dren keep their hands clean, too.
2. Keep countertops, cutting boards, and sinks clean. When preparing food, make sure all cooking surfaces have been washed well.

3. Use different and clean knives/utensils when preparing foods. Utensils that touch raw meats should never be used for cutting vegetables or other foods unless they have been thoroughly cleaned. Any serving platter or dish used for raw products should be cleaned well before using it for any other food. Especially keep this in mind when cooking outdoors: *never* put cooked foods back on a plate that was used to carry the raw foods.

4. Wash dirty sponges, cloths, and towels. Choose clean ones regularly.

5. Keep an eye on food dates. Products are stamped with a "sell by" or "use by" date. Discard any expired food products.

6. Test temperatures of cooked meats to be sure they are thoroughly cooked. Safe cooking temperatures are as follows:
   Beef, lamb, veal, pork: 160 degrees Fahrenheit
   Poultry, whole turkey, and chicken: 180 degrees Fahrenheit
   Poultry, chicken parts: 170 degrees Fahrenheit
   Egg dishes: 160 degrees Fahrenheit
   Leftovers: 165 degrees Fahrenheit
   (When checking the temperature, place the thermometer in the thickest part of the meat without touching the bone.)

7. Thaw frozen foods in the refrigerator or in the microwave. Keep raw foods from touching other foods in the refrigerator.

8. Freeze or refrigerate all perishable foods immediately upon returning from the supermarket.

9. Avoid eating meats, particularly ground beef, if the juices are red or pink. Test doneness with the thermometer.

10. Buy pasteurized dairy products and eggs. Avoid unpasteurized milk, juice, raw eggs, or mixtures made with raw eggs.

11. Store raw meat and fish products in the freezer. Fish can be kept in the refrigerator for up to 1 day, poultry and ground beef will keep up to 2 days, and red meat will keep up to 4 days.

12. Refrigerate or freeze any leftovers immediately.

FOODNOTE

Never take a chance with the safety of a food.

C = Choose Sensibly

• *Choose a diet that is low in saturated fat and cholesterol and moderate in total fat.* The problem here is, fat has gotten a bad rap. Fat is *not* a bad thing. We actually *need* to eat fat in our daily diet (although, maybe not as much as we currently eat!). Fats are necessary nutrients that help our bodies grow, build tissues, and transport important fats and fat-soluble vitamins through the body. All individuals, including children, should limit daily fat intake to 30 percent of total calories. This translates into:

If Your Daily Calories Are:	Limit Your Total Grams of Fat to: (30%)	Limit Your Total Calories from Fat to: (9 calories/gram)
1,500	50	450
1,800	60	540
2,000	67	600
2,500	83	750
2,700	90	810

However, the term "fats" encompass both saturated and unsaturated (polyunsaturated and monounsaturated) fats. *Saturated fats* are primarily found in foods that come from animals: milk, dairy products, meats, cheese, and ice cream, along with cakes, cookies, pastries, butter, and mayonnaise. These fats can impact a child's cholesterol level, which can increase incidence of heart disease, cancer, and obesity. So avoid saturated fats as much as possible. *Cholesterol,* a fatlike, waxy substance, is also primarily found in fats coming from animal sources. Foods that contain a lot of cholesterol are also typically high in saturated fats. These foods, too, are ones that need to be limited in the diet as they tend to raise blood cholesterol levels and can lead to future problems like heart attacks, strokes, or even some types of cancer.

Unsaturated fats are typically fats like vegetable oils and those found in some seafood. These fats *don't* cause cholesterol levels to rise and *don't* lead to heart problems, but can still have an impact on weight gain if eaten in excess. These are the better fats for you and your child.

• *Choose beverages and foods to moderate your intake of sugars.* Sugars are carbohydrates, too, but simple ones. Some of these sugars occur naturally in foods in the form of fructose, found in fruits and vegetables, and lactose in milk. Others, such as sucrose or table sugar, are added to make food sweeter either when the food is processed (soft drinks, sweetened cereals, packaged cookies, and the like), or prepared at home. As desirable as sugar may be, we suggest enjoying the good taste of natural sugars, like those in fruits, and limiting excess candies, cookies, cakes, and soft drinks.

• *Choose and prepare foods with less salt.* Salt is a combination of sodium and chloride, both important nutrients in our bodies. Salt helps with water balance in our body fluids and cells. Eating too much salt usually does not cause problems for children. But in adults, excess salt in the diet may cause water retention and problems with fluid balance and blood pressure. Thus learning to like salty foods at a young age may make it difficult to make necessary changes and reduce one's intake when older. Health problems associated with older individuals, such as hypertension (high blood pressure), heart disease, stroke, and kidney disease, often require a lower salt intake. Our best suggestion for most people, including children, is to enjoy the natural salt found in foods, but limit use of the salt shaker.

• *If you drink alcoholic beverages, do so in moderation.* As parents, we hope you take this into consideration. As alcohol is considered a drug and thereby unhealthy for children, we advise you to act as role models. If you do drink alcohol, do so with discretion.

Now you know the ABCs of planning and balancing your child's diet. Not an easy task, but if you use our guidelines it will make meal planning easier and will make your family's meals healthier.

3

A PRIMER ON NUTRIENTS
What We Get from Our Food

Did you know there are more than forty nutrients needed daily by our bodies? When we eat, our food moves through our digestive system, where it is broken down into nutrients that are absorbed into the bloodstream and carried to body cells. Of the nutrients, carbohydrates, protein, and fat supply us with energy (which is measured in calories). Our primary nutrients include:

• *Carbohydrates* supply us with our main source of energy. Whole grains, starches, pasta, milk, fresh fruits, and vegetables all contribute to this group. Carbohydrates provide 4 calories per gram of food, and should account for 50 to 55 percent of our daily calories.

• *Protein* provides the building blocks that keep our tissues, organs, and muscles healthy. Protein is primarily found in meat, eggs, beans, and dairy products. It also contributes 4 calories per gram of food, and should account for 15 to 20 percent of our daily calories.

• *Fat* gives us energy, helps our body grow, and is needed to transport important fat-soluble vitamins through the body. Aside from the obvious sources of fats—butter, margarine, oil, mayonnaise, and salad dressings—much of the fat we eat is "hidden" in our foods. For example, whole milk has more fat than skim milk, chicken with skin has more fat than skinless, and cheese is 80 percent fat. Other fat comes from the way we prepare our foods. For example, frying uses more fat than grilling, broiling, steaming, or poaching. Fat contributes over twice as many calories per gram of food than carbohydrates and protein at 9 calories per gram of food, and should account for up to 30 percent of daily calories.

• *Water*, though many people don't realize it, is a nutrient, and a very important one. Water regulates body temperature, carries nutrients to cells, and helps eliminate bodily wastes. Water makes up about 60 percent of our total body weight.

• *Vitamins and minerals, including vitamins A, C, and D, calcium, iron, and sodium,* come from a variety of foods found in the food pyramid. Some foods provide more of one kind of vitamin or mineral and others less. If children eat a well-balanced diet, with selections from all the food groups, they should get the variety of nutrients they need.

Our previous discussion on the Dietary Guidelines provided a detailed discussion on carbohydrates and fat. So here we will elaborate on our intake of protein, fiber, calcium, iron, and the antioxidant vitamins. (Note: Although fiber is not considered a nutrient, it is a vital component of a healthy diet.)

Meeting the Need for Protein

Many parents think their child just doesn't eat enough protein. Protein is essential for growth, development, and the workings of all body functions. Every part of our body—skin, muscle, bones, and organs—is made of protein.

FOODNOTE
The average person eats two times the requirement for protein.

But too *much* protein—and, of course, too *little* protein—is not advised. Current recommendations are .5 grams/pound for children seven to ten years of age unless the child is involved in very active sports. In this case, the requirement can edge upwards to .6 to .9 grams/pound. This translates to somewhere in the neighborhood of 40 to 50 grams of protein for the average 80 to 100-pound child. Children older than ten should begin to move toward the recommended dietary allowance of 46 grams/day for teen girls and 59 grams/day for teen boys.

RECOMMENDED DIETARY ALLOWANCES FOR PROTEIN

Age	Gender	RDA (grams)
7–10	boys and girls	28
11–18	girls	44–46
11–18	boys	45–59

Luckily, children 8 to 18 years of age usually meet their need for protein, as defined by the RDA. In fact, in the United States, protein is frequently eaten in excess because of the abundant sources and its good taste. Protein is found in foods like cheese, milk, yogurt, cottage cheese, eggs, meats, poultry, peanut butter, and tuna fish. These are very kid-friendly foods. Some protein is also found in such vegetables as dried beans and peas, soybeans, chickpeas, and lentils. However, protein-rich foods can also be high in saturated fat. Thus, it is wise to opt for lower-fat versions, choosing low-fat milk instead of whole milk; low-fat cheese and cottage cheese instead of regular; and ground sirloin or ground chuck instead of ground beef. Eating more protein than is needed does not benefit anyone: it just turns into body fat and puts extra stress on the kidneys and liver. Remember that no more than 15 to 20 percent of daily calories should come from protein. The following chart indicates some healthy protein sources.

Source of Protein	Serving Size	Amount of Protein (grams)
beef, poultry, fish, or pork	3 oz.	21
cottage cheese	½ cup	12
legumes, peas, or lentils	½ cup	9
milk—whole, 2%, or skim	8 oz.	8
yogurt	8 oz.	8
peanut butter	2 tablespoons	8
whole egg	1	7
egg white	1	3
bread, grains, or cereal	1 slice or 1 oz.	3
pasta or rice	½ to ¾ cup, cooked	3

How Much Fiber Is Enough?

Although not a nutrient, fiber is still a major component for a healthy diet. It's a fact that people of all ages *don't* get enough fiber in their diets. In some cases, the average person is eating less than *half* of what is needed.

Also referred to as roughage, dietary fiber is the part of grains, vegetables, fruit, beans, nuts, and seeds that cannot be digested by the body. There are two types of dietary fiber: insoluble and soluble. Both types are important in the diet. *Insoluble* fiber, which does not dissolve in water, is found in wheat and corn bran; whole wheat breads; cereals; some vegetables, such as cauliflower, green beans, and potatoes; and skins of fruits and root vegetables. Soluble fiber, which forms a gel-like substance and can dissolve in hot water, is found in most fruits and vegetables, such as apples, oranges, carrots, dried beans, peas, barley, and oats.

The body cannot actually digest fiber, so fiber helps move food through the intestine more quickly for better digestion. Additionally, it helps in forming stools, eliminating wastes, and reducing problems associated with constipation. Because high-fiber foods are more filling, they also are helpful in satisfying the appetite and preventing overeating.

A healthy adult should strive for 20 to 35 grams of fiber each day. A formula widely used by the American Dietetic Association and the American Academy of Pediatrics was developed to help children get amounts best suited for their particular age:

Child's age + 5 = amount of fiber recommended each day
Therefore:

a child who is 8 years old *needs:* $\quad$ 8 + 5 = *13* grams of fiber each day

a child who is 10 years old *needs:* $\quad$ 10 + 5 = *15* grams of fiber each day

a child who is 12 years old *needs:* $\quad$ 12 + 5 = *17* grams of fiber each day

a child who is 15 years old *needs:* $\quad$ 15 + 5 = *20* grams of fiber each day

Many children reject high-fiber foods because these foods feel bulky, grainy, and are not as soft as foods containing little or no fiber. So try to incorporate higher-fiber choices at a young age to allow children to get used to including these foods in their diet.

FOODNOTE

Just because wheat bread is dark in color doesn't guarantee that it is made from whole grains. Some food companies use burnt sugar, molasses, or other colorings to fool consumers. So, check the label. In order for the product to be labeled "whole grain," the first ingredient listed on the product must be whole wheat or other whole grain.

There's another plus to keep in mind if your child learns to eat high-fiber foods at a young age. Doing so helps keep these foods in the diet as years go on, and the benefits of having a high-fiber diet as an adult helps in reducing incidence of cancer, diabetes, and obesity. Starting this habit early on can prevent problems later in life.

But how do you find the foods with the most fiber? And, how do you know how much fiber they contain? Here's a chart that will help make the process easier.

Sources of Dietary Fiber	Amount of Fiber (grams)
Breads and Cereals	
all bran and 100% bran cereals (1 cup)	more than 8
40% bran and raisin bran cereals (1 cup)	4–5
other corn, wheat, or bran cereals (1 cup)	2–3
whole-wheat/whole-grain breads and rolls	1–2
Rice and Pasta	
brown or wild rice ($\frac{1}{2}$ cup)	2
barley or whole wheat pasta ($\frac{1}{2}$ cup)	2
Legumes	
cooked dried peas, beans, lentils ($\frac{1}{2}$ cup)	4–6
Fruits and Vegetables	
apple/pear without skin (1 medium)	2
apple/pear with skin	3
applesauce ($\frac{1}{2}$ cup)	2
banana (1 medium), blueberries ($\frac{1}{2}$ cup)	2
broccoli, spinach, carrots ($\frac{1}{2}$ cup)	2
raisins ($\frac{1}{3}$ cup), prunes (4), strawberries ($\frac{3}{4}$ cup)	3
baked potato with skin (1 medium)	4

FOODNOTE
A food is a good source of fiber if it has 2.5 grams/serving or more.

Calcium: Strengthen Those Bones!

Studies have shown that calcium intake before and during the adolescent years is extremely important. This is especially true for females, in order for them to reach their peak bone mass and protect against later incidence of osteoporosis.

FOODNOTE
Calcium keeps bones in shape—for a lifetime of use.

For years we heard our parents say, "drink your milk." Now many of us are saying this to *our* children. But do we know *why*? Milk is the primary source of calcium in the diet and a healthy beverage choice. When soft drinks replace milk at mealtime (and between meals, too), the amount of calcium consumed is significantly reduced.

Calcium is not only known to help build bones, it is also important for healthy heart muscles and blood. If you don't get enough calcium in your diet, your body will take it from your bones in order to supply its needs.

Up until twenty years of age, calcium requirements are 1,300 mg./day, because much calcium is absorbed by the bones. During preteen, teen, and young adult years, the body uses calcium for building bones and strengthening bone tissue. After this time, requirements are reduced to 1,000 mg./day, but we continue to need calcium in our diets. Somewhere around the age of thirty-five, the body stops adding to its existing bone mass. From this time on, many people begin to lose bone mass. This loss of bone mass is highly related to diet and exercise. Calcium intake during all of these years, along with regular exercise, can help prevent osteoporosis, a condition that strikes mainly older women, but also some men. It causes bones to become brittle and weak, and therefore easily broken. When bone density is decreased, or bones have not received adequate calcium through the years, this condition is more likely to occur.

The most important time to set the stage for building adequate bone mass and following an adequate exercise program is during the childhood and teen years. In preteen and teenage girls who may follow extreme weight loss diets or may be prone to eating disorders, bone mass can be highly affected. In fact, in extreme cases, bone disease can *begin* in adolescence. Also, children who spend large amounts of time in front of the television or computer are prone to obesity, and their bone growth may suffer from immobilization and lack of exercise as well.

In the preteen and teen years, children make more of their own food choices, and may tend to choose greater amounts of high-fat and high-sodium foods and snacks, or to follow fad diets. These extreme choices can affect overall bone mass. Large amounts of sodium (salt) and phosphates (from soft drinks) in a diet can inhibit calcium deposits in bones. Parents need to keep a watchful eye on their children's intake and activities during this important growth period. A balanced food intake along with a mix of individual and team sports encourages overall benefits in bone strength and cardiovascular conditioning.

Milk and dairy products such as cheese, cottage cheese, ice cream, and yogurt are high in calcium. But, because they can also be high in fat, it's best to choose lower-fat versions of these foods. Other good sources of calcium include canned salmon and sardines; fortified orange juice; tofu; dark green leafy vegetables, such as kale, spinach, and broccoli; and cooked dried beans.

Source of Calcium	Serving Size	Amount of Calcium (mg)
low-fat milk	1 cup	300
low-fat chocolate milk	1 cup	280
skim milk powder	$\frac{1}{4}$ cup	400
low-fat ricotta cheese	$\frac{1}{2}$ cup	335
mozzarella cheese, part skim	1 oz.	260
cheddar cheese	1 oz.	205
low-fat cottage cheese	$\frac{1}{2}$ cup	75
low-fat yogurt	1 cup	400
low-fat frozen yogurt	$\frac{1}{2}$ cup	140
ice cream	$\frac{1}{2}$ cup	90
broccoli, cooked	1 cup	180

FOODNOTE
80 to 90 percent of girls and 60 to 70 percent of boys do *not* get adequate amounts of calcium in their diets.

Remember, the body *needs* calcium. It is important for you, as a parent, to try to get enough calcium into your child's diet. Foods should be the primary source of calcium, but if for some reason this is not possible, check with your doctor regarding the recommendation for a supplement.

Iron: For Strong, Healthy Blood

Iron plays an extremely important role in the body—yet amazingly, the total amount of iron in the body only adds up to about one teaspoonful.

Most of the iron in the body is found in the blood, particularly in the hemoglobin. Hemoglobin helps red blood cells carry oxygen from the lungs to the cells throughout the body, and carry carbon dioxide from body tissues back to the lungs for excretion. When iron supplies become depleted or the diet does not provide enough iron, an iron deficiency or anemia can occur. Iron-deficiency anemia is common during teen years, particularly among females. This is due to the increased growth spurt that occurs during these years, the loss of blood that occurs during monthly menstrual periods, and the typically smaller amounts of food that girls eat. If your teenager is athletic, this adds to the need for increased iron, as iron is lost in perspiration.

The recommended intake of iron for males and females seven to ten years old is 10 mg./day. Preteen and teenage boys need 12 mg./day. Following age eighteen, this requirement for males goes back to 10 mg./day largely because the body has stopped growing. Girls, on the other hand, lose blood each month when they menstruate, so their requirements during preteen and teen years are higher at 15 mg./day. They continue to need 15 mg./day on into adulthood.

Lean red meat, seafood, egg yolks, legumes, dried beans, nuts, dark green leafy vegetables, fortified grain, and cereal products are all good dietary sources of iron. The many enriched and fortified food products available in today's market will definitely add to your total iron intake and that of your child.

The following chart shows the iron content of various common foods. One fact to remember is that the body's iron absorption is better and more efficient from animal food sources than from plant sources. In addition, ascorbic acid, also known as vitamin C, helps the absorption of iron. So, if you eat or drink a vitamin C source with your iron-containing food item, the iron will be better absorbed. For example, if you drink a glass of orange juice when you eat an iron-fortified cereal, the iron from the cereal will be absorbed by the body more efficiently.

Source of Iron	Portion Size	Amount of Iron (mg.)
lean sirloin, broiled	3 oz.	2.9
lean ground beef	3 oz.	1.8
chicken, dark meat	3 oz.	1.1
chicken, white meat	3 oz.	1.0
lean pork	3 oz.	1.0
canned salmon	3 oz.	.7
fortified cereal	1 cup	4.5–18.0
soybean nuts	½ cup	4.0
beans/legumes	½ cup	2.5
raisins	⅓ cup	1.1
prunes	5	1.1
peanut butter	2 tablespoons	.6
bread, fortified	1 slice	.7–.9
enriched rice	½ cup	1.2

The Antioxidant Vitamins: Why They Can Be So Important

Several vitamins, such as vitamins C, E, and beta-carotene (a form of vitamin A), are classified as *antioxidant vitamins,* and are known to reduce the risk of cancer and other diseases in the body. These vitamins are abundantly found in a variety of fruits and vegetables, and can assist in improving overall health and resistance to disease in one's later years.

Many foods at the supermarket are fortified with antioxidants. While they might not provide enough vitamins for protective benefits, they do contain sources of these nutrients. Ultimately fruits and vegetables are still the best sources of vitamin C and beta-carotene, and they may also provide protective compounds against health problems like cancer and heart disease later in life.

The word is still out on the benefit of taking antioxidants in the form of a dietary supplement. Until further research is completed, our best advice to you and your children is to stick with eating fruits, vegetables, and grains with naturally occurring antioxidants.

There's a lot that goes into keeping our kids strong and healthy. Providing a variety of foods is one way you, as a parent, can meet this goal. The many vitamins, minerals, and other key nutrients needed to attain optimum growth and development are more likely to be obtained with a diversified selection of foods. The younger children are when they begin to eat healthfully, the greater their chances of living a longer, better quality life.

4

SHOULD I BE CONCERNED?
Caffeine, Artificial Sweeteners, Fat Replacers, Dietary Supplements, and Other Food Safety Issues

Children and teens are often influenced by new food and nutrition trends. Because of the media, their peers, and/or family members, our younger generation is on the move to try new products. The coffee bar explosion, along with the pressure to be a super athlete or stick-thin, has brought our kids to seek out caffeine, food replacers, and dietary supplements more than ever before. Here's a rundown on these issues and their effect on children today.

Caffeine and Caffeine Products

Caffeine is part of a group of compounds called *methylxanthines* that are naturally found in many products like coffee and cocoa beans, cola nuts, and tea leaves. When thinking about caffeine and its effects, adults typically think of coffee as its primary source in the diet. But for children, soft drinks are the number one contributing source of caffeine.

Caffeine is a *drug*. It is an addictive stimulant that directly affects the nervous system, kidneys, and other body systems. Although caffeine does not accumulate in the body and is eventually excreted, it can still cause increased energy levels, alertness, and increased mental abilities especially within the first hour after consumption.

However, excess caffeine consumption can cause a person to be fidgety, inattentive, and easily distracted. These symptoms often mimic those of Attention Deficit Disorder/Attention Deficit Hyperactive Disorder (ADD/ADHD). Because of this, many parents rush to the conclusion that their child may suffer from ADD/ADHD symptoms and seek medication to control the problem. If your child exhibits these symptoms, it may be wise for you or your pediatrician to evaluate whether the cause could be caffeine-related.

Adults typically consume 200 mg. of caffeine/day, primarily in the form of coffee. Children aged eight to eighteen who get their caffeine from soft drinks, teas, and chocolate should consume no more than 25 to 50 mg. caffeine daily. As a parent, first unobtrusively monitor how much caffeine your child may be getting, and then attempt to correct the situation should the intake be high.

Source of Caffeine	Serving Size	Amount of Caffeine (mg)
coffee, brewed	8 oz.	60–180
coffee, instant	8 oz.	30–120
coffee, decaffeinated	8 oz.	1–5
tea, brewed	8 oz.	20–90
tea, iced	8 oz.	9–50
soft drinks	8 oz.	20–40
chocolate, milk	1 oz.	1–15
chocolate, dark	1 oz.	5–35
chocolate, semi-sweet	1 oz.	5–35
chocolate syrup	1 oz.	4
chocolate milk	8 oz.	2–7

FOODNOTE

To reduce caffeine levels, try caffeine-free soft drinks (in moderation, of course) and beverages like lemonade, 100% fruit juice, and—best yet—water.

Artificial Sweeteners and Fat Replacers

Artificial Sweeteners

Artificial sweeteners have been available to consumers for years. Initially, they were marketed to people who could not metabolize sugar in the bloodstream. Today, food producers have flooded food products with artificial sweeteners to help entice consumers eat less sugar in their diets. With greater sweetening power than table sugar, these sweeteners sweeten foods as well as reduce or eliminate calories.

FOODNOTE

Sugar contains 16 calories per teaspoon as compared to artificial sweeteners, which contain 0 to 2 calories per teaspoon.

Scientists are continually investigating potential hazards associated with the use of artificial sweeteners. To date, no scientific evidence has shown artificial sweeteners to present problems as long as they are used in reasonable amounts. Although some people report such side effects as dizziness, headaches, or nausea after consuming foods with artificial sweeteners, the Food and Drug Administration considers these sweeteners to be safe to consume. Information is provided on food labels to allow consumers to make informed decisions about the foods they choose. But just to be safe, let's take a close look at the three most popular calorie-free artificial sweeteners.

1. Aspartame

Commercially known as Equal and NutraSweet, aspartame has been available to consumers for over twenty years. It is primarily used to sweeten fat-free sweet foods, such as ice cream, cookies, and diet soft drinks.

Aspartame is made from two amino acids (phenylalanine and aspartic acid). When these two substances are put together they form a compound that is *200 times* as sweet as sugar! Because of this increased sweetening power, less aspartame is needed to sweeten foods, therefore reducing overall calories.

Many people believe that aspartame is bad, particularly for children, because of the controversy over how aspartame breaks down in the body. Yet researchers to date have found no evidence of any short- or long-term problems associated with moderate amounts of aspartame in the diet.

Warning: Some children may be sensitive or allergic to aspartame and may experience discomfort, such as headaches or stomachaches, after eating foods containing it. Others may not be able to metabolize the amino acid found in aspartame, phenylalanine, because they have an ailment called Phenylketonuria or PKU. PKU is usually diagnosed in infancy, and your doctor should have told you if this is a concern for your child. PKU children should avoid use of aspartame altogether, and products containing aspartame must be labeled to indicate that they contain phenylalanine.

2. Acesulfame K (Sunette)

This sweetener became available in the late 1980s and is used in many prepared foods. Also *200 times* as sweet as sugar, Acesulfame K contributes no calories to foods because the body does not digest it. As it has a slight aftertaste, it is commonly used in combination with other sweeteners and is found in chewing gums, powdered drink mixes, puddings, baked goods, frozen desserts, and nondairy creamers.

3. Saccharin

The oldest of all artificial sweeteners, saccharin is *300 times* as sweet as sugar. Some consumers shy away from using saccharin because of studies that claim saccharin causes cancer in laboratory animals. In fact, products containing saccharin used to require this statement on their label: "Use of this product may be hazardous to your health. This product contains saccharin, which has been determined to cause cancer in laboratory animals."

Recent legislation was passed to eliminate this requirement, because no ill effects are known to exist from consuming products that contain saccharin. Many recommend a moderate intake of products containing saccharin for adults and children alike.

Fat Replacers

With all the hype about cutting dietary fat, food manufacturers continue to scramble to find a good-tasting fat substitute that can easily be used in foods. So new fat-free products are filling our supermarket shelves daily—some tasty, others not!

Unfortunately, no fat substitute has it all. Some cannot stand up to high cooking temperatures, while others can't be fried, frozen, or stored at room temperature. It's very difficult to make a duplicate for real fat, especially one that tastes good, looks good, feels good, and fulfills our desire for fat.

Simplesse, a protein-based fat substitute; Olestra, a fat-based fat substitute; and Oatrim, a carbohydrate-based fat substitute, have all been used in different food products.

Derived from egg-white protein or milk protein, *Simplesse* is used in cheese, ice cream, salad dressing, and mayonnaise. Because it breaks down when exposed to heat, this substitute primarily is used in cold foods.

Olestra is a fat-based fat substitute made from vegetable oils that can be heated, and is most often used in corn chips, potato chips, and tortilla chips. Many scientists thought this would be the ultimate answer to the fat-substitute problem, as Olestra possesses all the properties of normal fat, but is made into a larger molecule that passes through the digestive system without being absorbed and digested. However, public action groups have fought against its release and use because they believe this substance could have long-term health effects on many people. Since it is not absorbed into the body, they claim that the absorption of important fat-soluble vitamins (A, D, E, and K) is also blocked. Additional complaints of stomachaches, cramping, and diarrhea have led consumers to be leery of and less interested in using products with Olestra. Until further long-term studies on children and young adults are completed, many people feel that children should limit their intake of this fat substitute.

Carbohydrate-based fat substitutes are also moving into the food supply. One such example, *Oatrim,* is made from a combination of modified food starches incorporating oat flour and oat bran. These substances can be used in baking, but not frying, and are currently being used in baked goods, salad dressings, and ice cream.

Seeking a fat replacement in the diet is not all that it is made out to be, especially as fats are important in the diet for proper growth and development and maintaining overall good health. Fats help absorb fat-soluble vitamins and contribute to energy needs, particularly in young and active children.

FOODNOTE

Fat replacers can reduce the amount of fat consumed only if fat is limited at other meals and throughout the day.

Parents should keep in mind that sugar substitutes and fat substitutes are not always the best choices when it comes to feeding their children. Each has its particular place in our food supply and can be useful when consumed in *moderate* amounts. But many consumers believe that these substitutes are the answer to our problems with excess eating, that with the use of these products we can eat all we want and not worry about the consequences. In fact, the opposite can occur: when consumed in excess amounts, these products can be more harmful than helpful. *Moderation* is the key. Our society as a whole has not gotten slimmer, but has gotten more overweight since it has been introduced to the wide variety of low-fat, low-sugar products.

Dietary Supplements: What They Are and What They Do

Dietary supplements are a booming business these days and getting bigger all the time. Reports indicate that more than half of the adult population currently uses some type of supplement on a regular basis. It is important for parents to ask: *What kind of message is this giving to our children? How are supplements affecting our dietary habits?*

Dietary supplements used to be a multivitamin/mineral tablet, taken once a day, that supplemented the diet with 100 percent of the Recommended Dietary Allowance. Parents often chose to give their children a fruit-flavored, cartoon character pill just to ensure that they would be getting what they needed each day. No longer is this the case. Dietary supplements now available have expanded from adding an extra boost of vitamins and minerals to those that include all types of herbs and botanicals. These products come in tablets, pills, powders, and liquids, and are being sold by health food stores, mall kiosks, supermarkets, mail order catalogs, individual salespersons, and even over the Internet. Many of these supplements claim various health benefits, pain relief, energy boosts, time-released formulas, longevity, and much more. Can these supplements and other products be trusted? Are they safe? Are they supported and approved by our government agencies? And, *does your child need to take a supplement?* Let's look at the answers to these questions.

Vitamin/mineral/fiber and other nutrient supplements are commonly available to people of all ages. But are they really *necessary?* Individuals that eat a varied diet do not usually need daily vitamin/mineral supplements. Supplements cannot, and do not, supply all the substances needed for good health. In large quantities, they can often be toxic and dangerous. We believe that there's no need to give our children supplements if they seem to be eating a varied diet.

However, special circumstances do require supplements at various stages of a person's life. These would include pregnancy; old age; and any food intolerance, allergy, or nutrient deficiency. In children and teens, most common are iron deficiency anemia and a lack of calcium due to lactose intolerance. Just bear in mind that *the use of supplements on a regular basis cannot substitute for the importance of healthy food choices and a proper diet.*

The Food and Drug Administration (FDA) is responsible for regulating drugs. As dietary supplements are not classified as drugs, the FDA does *not* monitor the use or safety of these products. While federal laws do require manufacturers to ensure that their products are safe before they are marketed to the public, it is up to individual consumers to understand and research products they use for safety, effectiveness, and health. If consumers are uninformed, as the case may be with teenagers or younger children, selecting the wrong product could be dangerous. Parents also can be uninformed or misinformed. It is your responsibility as a parent to know what you give your children and what they are taking themselves.

Many young athletes are drawn to dietary aids and supplements, believing that these products will enhance performance. *Children need to understand that no supplement of any type can compete with a balanced diet, good training, and hard work.* Consider the messages you relay to your child regarding supplements of any type: Children are more encouraged to try and to use these products if their parents do so. And, when these behaviors begin at a young age, they likely continue into the future.

FOODNOTE

Multivitamins are meant to enhance the diet, not replace foods that should be eaten. That's why they are referred to as "supplements."

Controversies surround the use of health benefits and claims on labels that accompany dietary supplements. Manufacturers rely on these to help sell their products—but can we trust these statements? Under current laws and regulations, manufacturers of supplements can use the following claims:

• *Nutrient-content claims* identify the level of a particular nutrient in the supplement with a statement about its benefits. Example: "This product contains 10 mg. vitamin C per serving and is a good source of vitamin C."

• *Disease claims* identify the connection between the supplement and a health condition. Example: "This product is high in calcium, which is known to help build strong bones."

• *Nutrition-support claims* identify a connection between the supplement and a deficiency disease. Example: "This product contains vitamin C, which is known to prevent the disease scurvy."

Consumers should always be on their guard for fraudulent claims. There are so many products available—some are a waste of money and others are even harmful to our health. Keep a watchful eye for products that may seem too good to be true. Claims like "miracle cure," "magical product," and "instant success" should immediately bring up a red flag of caution.

Diet supplements encompass a wide range of products, including vitamins, minerals, herbs, amino acids, steroids, and weight loss/gain items. They are found in tablet, capsule, or liquid form. Here are a few examples of the types of dietary supplements that you or your child may encounter that you need to be aware of.

• *Amino acids* are supplements often used by athletes to build muscles and increase fat loss. Teenagers who are active in sports and muscle building may be tempted to use amino acids. Generally, most athletes get more than enough amino acids in their diet. Excessive protein in the form of amino acids is unnecessary and may put stress on the kidneys and liver to filter the excess out of the body, possibly causing permanent damage.

• *Carnitine* is made of two amino acids: lysine and methionine. It is used by athletes as an ergogenic aid, that is, to provide more energy, power, and reduce body fat. Athletic teens are eager to try this supplement. Evidence of supplemental benefits is unavailable at this time. There is really no need to take carnitine as a supplement, as the body produces adequate amounts and a diet that includes meat contains plenty of carnitine.

• *Ginseng,* a plant root, is promoted to improve the sex drive and as a cure-all for numerous ailments from memory loss to stress to chronic pains. To date, there has been no scientific evidence able to prove these benefits. Taken over time, ginseng has been shown to cause detrimental side effects such as alterations in blood pressure, sleep loss, anxiety, sedative effects, and vaginal bleeding.

• *Chromium picolinate* is used by athletes as an ergogenic and weight loss aid. Teenagers are drawn to it for these reasons. Chromium is a part of insulin, and works in the body to produce energy. There is no evidence that extra chromium produces extra energy or provides any added benefits. Supplements usually provide higher than recommended levels and may be harmful.

• *Creatine phosphate* is used by athletes as an ergogenic aid to promote energy and increase endurance. Teen athletes are lured to creatine for these reasons. As the body makes creatine in adequate amounts, taking a supplement does not seem warranted. Research at this time has not proven supplemental benefits.

• *Lecithin* is a type of fat that has been hailed to cure or prevent arthritis, skin problems, gallstones, and nervous disorders. Claims have also been made that it can dissolve fat on our body and cholesterol in the arteries. Your body makes lecithin. Therefore, taking additional lecithin does not seem necessary. Synthetic lecithin is absorbed poorly by the body.

• *Medicinal herbs* Depending on the product, the effects of the herbs will be different. Herbs, such as chamomile, echinacea, ginger, garlic, and valerian may have beneficial physical effects, but currently there is not enough information to make a recommendation for their use, especially with children and teens. On the other hand, there may be some dangers from taking herbs in combination with some medications. It's best to consult your doctor before using any herbal product.

• *Ma Huang,* also called ephedra, is an herb taken to promote energy and help with weight loss. Taken for too long or used improperly, ma huang can be dangerous, causing high blood pressure, increased heart rate, muscle injury, and nerve damage. These side effects would definitely be reasons our children and teenagers should not use this supplement. Consult your doctor before using ma huang.

• *Steroids* appeal to teen athletes because of their reputation as muscle-building enhancers. Steroids are drugs and are made to act like the male hormone testosterone. While they may build bigger muscles, steroids have not been shown to necessarily improve athletic performance. More important are the dangers of taking steroids. In men, steroids can cause acne, lower sperm count, damage the testes, and enlarge breasts. In women, steroids often cause a lower voice, facial hair, smaller breasts, and irregularity of or cessation of menstrual cycles. Building muscle through physical training and hard work is still the best approach.

• *High potency vitamins and minerals* are any tablets, capsules, or pills that supply vitamins or minerals in excessive amounts, as compared to the Recommended Dietary Allowances (RDAs). There are no government regulations limiting the strength of most vitamins and minerals. Therefore, the strength of vitamin/mineral supplements on the market could be greater than what most people, and especially children and teens, need. Excessive intake of most vitamins and minerals can be harmful and may cause fatigue, headaches, diarrhea, and hair loss as well as more serious side effects, such as kidney stones and kidney damage; liver, bone, or nerve damage; birth defects; or even death. *More* is not always better. A healthy, well-balanced diet is still the best way to go.

• *Over-the-counter diet aids and appetite suppressants.* Several appetite suppressants and diet aids are available on the market today and are approved by the FDA for short-term use, that is, a few weeks or months. However, there are no regulatory controls in place to monitor how long people stay on these products. No studies have been done regarding the effects or safety of diet aids/appetite suppressants on children and/or teens. Our recommendation is for children and teenagers *not* to use these items. In addition, we suggest that parents, who act as role models, not use them, either. Remember, these products can be *addictive*.

As we look into what the future holds for dietary supplements, it is clear that demand will indeed bring on the supply. People of all ages are drawn to these products, and as long as sales are up, more and more choices will become available.

Parents need to be educated on what's hot, what's available, and what other kids are talking about. Products claiming to help lose weight, build muscle, increase your stamina, and keep you alert will be ones that attract the younger generation. As anyone can walk into a store and purchase these products, keep on top of your children's concerns, and help them find better solutions. For example, if your teen feels the need to lose weight and desires to purchase a canned or powdered weight loss supplement, it may be better to seek the advice of your doctor or registered dietitian first. Better safe than sorry.

FOODNOTE

There's no greater benefit to health than a healthy diet.

Other Food Safety Issues

How safe *is* our food? Food safety issues are a major concern for parents and children alike. Our newspapers and other media are filled with stories of people eating contaminated foods. In reality, most cases of food poisoning are not life-threatening, but they can cause very unpleasant symptoms, such as stomachaches, diarrhea, nausea, headaches, and vomiting. As a parent, how can you make sure your family's food is safe? What current and new forms of technology exist that help improve the safety of our food? Are organic foods better for you? Are raw foods safe to eat?

Pesticides

The Environmental Protection Agency (EPA) defines pesticides as substances that protect food from any pests, including insects, rodents, weeds, molds, and bacteria.

When we think of pesticides, we generally think of synthetic chemicals. However, there are naturally occurring chemicals, such as copper, sulfur, and nicotine, that are also used. New forms of pest control are in development to make our food supply safe and plentiful.

The EPA constantly studies the levels of pesticides used to keep our food supplies safe for adults as well as for children. Health professionals believe that pesticides used on crops keep them safe and that consumers should continue to eat these fruits and vegetables in their diet. Chances are good that without pesticide use farmers could not produce the amount and quality of crops they currently produce. The benefits of eating these foods far outweigh any risks attributed to potential pesticide residues. But, to be safe, all food should be washed thoroughly before eating.

Foodborne Illnesses

Basically, foodborne illnesses are caused as a result of organisms contaminating foods. Primarily these organisms are bacterial. Most forms of foodborne illness are mild and only last several hours, although some forms can be more critical. Children, pregnant women, and seniors particularly can be more susceptible to a more serious infection.

The following is a list of common forms of organisms that can contaminate our food. We've included the foods they are likely to effect, as well as the symptoms of the foodborne illnesses they cause.

- *Staphylococcus* is primarily found in meats, poultry, egg products, tuna, potato and macaroni salads, and cream-filled pastries stored at room temperature. Symptoms usually occur within two to six hours after ingestion and include diarrhea, vomiting, nausea, and cramping. Symptoms usually subside within one to three days.

- *Salmonella* is commonly associated with eggs and egg products such as mayonnaise, undercooked poultry, meat, dairy products, seafood, and fresh produce and foods not properly refrigerated. Symptoms usually occur within six to forty-eight hours after ingestion and include vomiting, nausea, cramping, diarrhea, fever, headache, and occasionally a rash. These infections can sometimes be serious, especially in infants, young children, and seniors.

- *Clostridium botulinum* is found in improperly produced canned foods and foods that have a low acid content, such as green beans, mushrooms, spinach, olives, and beef. Symptoms usually occur within twelve to thirty-six hours. Botulism directly affects the nervous system, and can be quite serious, causing paralysis and even death. Be sure to avoid any foods that have a suspicious odor or canned foods that appear to have been damaged.

- *E. Coli* is associated with undercooked beef, unpasteurized milk, lettuce, untreated water, unpasteurized fruit juices, and any food handed without washing hands, particularly after changing diapers and using the bathroom. Symptoms usually include cramping and diarrhea, which may escalate to a more severe situation depending on the individual case, and can even be fatal in young children.

Most forms of foodborne illness are preventable with some simple methods of storing, handling, and preparing foods, especially at home. It just takes some food safety precautions to keep your food safe for everyone to eat (see the Food Safety Guide in chapter 2).

Irradiation

Have you heard about irradiation yet? It sounds sort of scary, yet you may be seeing more foods moving into the supermarket with labels indicating that they have been treated by irradiation.

Irradiation is a process of treating foods to help prevent contamination. It's a type of cold pasteurization, using gamma rays to kill any bacteria or fungi in the food. This low level of radiation helps reduce the risk of contamination and keep the food perfectly safe to eat. It also helps increase the food product's shelf life, improves the quality of fresh foods, and can replace the use of chemical preservatives. Spices and seasonings have undergone irradiation treatments since the early 1960s. Currently the Food and Drug Administration allows foods containing wheat flour, poultry, pork, and some fruits and vegetables to be treated with irradiation. Approval for fish, seafood, ground beef, and processed meats should take place in the near future.

Irradiated foods will taste and look the same as they did before. But they must be labeled so consumers can choose to buy these foods or not. Keep in mind that food processors are aiming to make our food supply safer, so consumers should not be afraid to eat foods that have been proven to be safe. But, as safe as these foods are, they do not replace safety measures for food preparation (see the Food Safety Guide in chapter 2).

FOODNOTE

Food processors are continually aiming to make our foods safer. We should not be afraid of new technology.

Biotechnology and Genetically Modified Foods

Food reengineering or genetic modification refers to the process of growing or breeding crops to create a specific trait. Examples of such crops are soybeans or potatoes that resist pest infestation and tomatoes that will not ripen too quickly. This technology can improve the way a food is grown as well as improve its taste once it reaches your plate.

Biotechnology can be a useful way to make the best use out of declining farms, especially considering the large number of people that need to be fed. The potential for higher yields and the reduction of pesticide and herbicide use will probably lead us to use this technology more and more.

Foods that have been genetically engineered will most likely not be labeled as such. But these foods are safe for us to eat: Their composition and nutritional value are basically the same as the traditional food (unless that specific trait is supposed to be altered).

Biotechnology in years to come may include the following:

- Fruits and vegetables grown with higher levels of vitamins C and E and beta-carotene.
- Potatoes grown with a higher starch content, which, because they would absorb less oil, could lead to lower-fat French fries and potato chips.
- New food varieties such as broccoflower.
- Foods known to trigger allergies modified to include fewer allergy-causing proteins.
- Crops developed to resist severe weather conditions and diseases.

FOODNOTE

Consumers need to be comfortable with the food choices they make. They need to keep up-to-date on food technology to understand what is being offered to them and what they are eating.

Organic Foods: A Better Choice?

Organic foods include fruits, vegetables, and meats that have been grown or raised without the use of synthetic pesticides, herbicides, hormones, or chemicals. Natural fertilizers, such as manure, are allowed to be used. Some people believe organic foods are safer and healthier to eat than conventional products. This is an individual decision; as yet, no scientific studies have proven they are healthier or safer than other foods.

Both organic and conventional farming methods can produce healthy crops. However, while well intended, organic farming alone cannot supply enough food for large populations, as it requires a great deal of care to produce organic crops.

As of 1998, the Organic Foods Production Act specifies consistent standards must be met to label a food "organically grown." The food must be certified by the U.S. Department of Agriculture and must have at least 50 percent of its ingredients produced organically. The food cannot contain any nitrates, nitrites, or sulfites.

Food Additives and Preservatives

Food additives include natural and synthetic components commonly added to our food supply. They offer you the ability to eat safe, wholesome foods year round. But you may notice the ingredient label on a food product and get nervous about unfamiliar names and additives listed. This may give you cause for concern about the foods you and your family are eating.

Additives used today are added to foods to improve the safety and nutritional quality, as well as improving the taste and appearance of the product. Some additives are so familiar, you may not even consider them "additives or preservatives." Salt and sugar are common additives, as well as vitamin D added to milk, and calcium added to orange juice.

All food additives are highly regulated by the U.S. Food and Drug Administration. Federal laws require that all substances be safe before they can be added to any food. Even after their introduction, they are continually monitored for safety.

The use of preservatives in foods also causes concern. Unless you plan on growing all of your own food and making everything from scratch, it is virtually impossible in today's world to eat foods without preservatives. The FDA monitors the safety of preservatives in foods, making sure the food in the marketplace is of high quality and safe to eat.

Preservatives are used to keep foods from spoiling, growing moldy, changing color, or becoming rancid. Food manufacturers add preservatives to help keep foods safe during transportation, during shelf life at the supermarket, and at home. Common types of preservatives include:

- *nitrites* to inhibit bacterial growth, enhance flavor and/or color
- *sulfites* to prevent or reduce discoloration in fruits and vegetables, and inhibit bacterial growth
- *BHA* (butylated hydroxyanisole) to reduce odor, discoloration, and flavor changes caused by exposure to air

---

FOODNOTE:

The wax on fruit is safe to eat. But washing is recommended before eating to remove any dirt, bacteria, or pesticide residue.

There's nothing wrong with buying foods made without preservatives. Always check the expiration date and look for spoilage. If you choose to use foods that are preservative-free, we suggest shopping more frequently, refrigerating well, and being more aware of cleanliness and thorough cooking methods.

Raw Foods

Popular trends of eating more raw fish, like sushi, and raw meat, like steak tartar, make some people worry about foodborne illness. It is very important to know and trust your source of raw fish and meat, if you choose to eat these foods, as there is a risk associated with eating these products. It's extremely important for your food source to follow strict sanitation standards and to only sell fresh fish and meat. Also, keep in mind that it is safer to eat sushi that is made with smoked fish, cooked fish, and/or vegetables.

Trying to understand and meet our own nutrition needs is difficult enough, but as parents we are responsible for the needs of our children as well. So much information is available, that it's just a matter of finding the right information and applying it. Here we have tried to supply you with a foundation on nutrition for healthy, active, growing children. Further sections of the book will help you to apply this information to specific concerns you may have regarding your child and to implement your foodsmarts to make the best choices for you and your family.

PART TWO

NUTRITION SOLUTIONS FOR YOUR CHILD

5

MY CHILD EATS TOO MUCH!
Helping the Overweight Child

Help! My child keeps gaining weight. Kids are teasing him. He won't listen to me when I tell him what to eat and what not to eat. What should I do?

Are these comments familiar? They are all too often heard from parents struggling with their overweight children. Since today's kids are becoming fatter and less active, and are adapting unhealthy lifestyles, obesity is on the rise.

Prevention is the key. As an overweight child grows older, his or her chances of becoming an obese adult increase. Think about it: The longer unhealthy habits exist, the stronger and more ingrained they become. By delaying or slowing excess weight gain during the pre-adolescent years, chances are you will help limit future weight gain problems for your child.

Obesity has both genetic and environmental causes and, currently, nothing has been found that can alter our genetic heritage. It's true that if both parents are overweight, a child has a 90 percent chance of becoming overweight. (The odds are less if only one parent is overweight.) However, it is not uncommon for siblings from the same parents to have different weight issues. Families often have one child who tends to be overweight and has to limit food selections, and one child who is underweight and needs to eat large quantities of food to put on weight. Which genes are inherited by your offspring just seems to depend on the luck of the draw.

Yet heredity should not be used as an *excuse* for obesity. Does a child gain too much weight just because of an inherited tendency to be overweight, or is it because eating and exercise habits are modeled after the people he or she lives with and the type of foods that are available and eaten in the house? Yes, it's also true that one's *environment* plays a key role in weight gain.

Besides, today's generation of children is more sedentary than ever before. Too much time is spent watching TV and playing video and computer games—activities that were not available when today's parents were growing up. If your child spends more than three hours a day at sedentary activities, it's too much; get him or her involved in sports and physical activities. Even better, join your child in these activities.

What other trends in our society lead to obesity in kids? Frequent eating away from home, greater availability of convenience foods, higher-fat snacks and junk foods, and increased consumption of non-nutritive, highly sugared beverages—all added to the decrease in physically activity—has caused more calories to be consumed than are being expended. Not surprisingly, our kids are becoming fat.

So many meals eaten away from home are eaten in fast food restaurants, malls, and school cafeterias. Complex carbohydrates and fiber, found in fruits, vegetables, and whole grains, are offered at a minimum at these places. It's more of the high-fat and high-sugar foods that are abundantly available. The problem is that while fat makes food taste good, it has twice the amount of calories as carbohydrates and protein. And since fruits and vegetables are not readily available when eating out, kids will eat more of the fattier foods because they are available and they taste good. These trends form habits—habits that stick, habits that are hard to break. Your children will automatically start reaching for the fried chicken or bag of chips rather than the banana or apple.

So it is important for you to set limits when eating out. (We will discuss this further in Part Three). But for now, think about choosing restaurants that offer healthier choices for your child, or packing healthy lunches rather than having him or her always buy school lunches. It also helps to have fruits and vegetables available and ready to snack on at home. While it's true that your kids are not going to pick healthy meals and snacks all of the time, encouraging healthier selections and making these options readily available at home *and* away from home may help your child make better choices overall.

Drinking lots of fruit drinks and soft drinks has also become a popular trend. These drinks provide calories and little else; essentially they offer only calories, an unhealthy option for anyone. An excessive intake of juice, even if it is 100% fruit juice, is not suggested either. Besides, juice and soft drinks do not quench thirst, as they are so highly concentrated with sugar. Drinking water is the healthiest way to take away thirst. Water is calorie-free, a necessary nutrient, and very refreshing. Six to eight glasses of water each day is ideal for most preteens and teens, although this is often difficult to attain. Keep in mind that many foods like soups, and fruits and vegetables can also contribute to our fluid needs.

Milk, as well as 100% fruit juice that has been fortified with calcium needed for building strong bones and teeth, needs to be consumed in the right amount to meet nutrient needs, and should not be considered as thirst quenchers. Three to four glasses of lower-fat milk or dairy products are recommended daily. There are no recommended allowances for fruit juices. Although they do contribute to your daily fruit requirement, they should not replace any more than two fruit servings a day.

It is difficult to combat obesity in your child. That is why it is so important to establish healthy habits when your children are young. Provide a variety and balance of foods; prepare healthy meals; establish healthy portion limitations; and set good eating and exercise examples for your children when they are toddlers. If your child is older, implement these same guidelines as soon as possible. Healthier habits are more difficult to establish the older one becomes, but be consistent and persistent. It *will* happen.

WHAT'S A PARENT TO DO?

- *Be a model yourself* by eating healthy, being active, and not constantly focusing on appearance.
- *Be positive.* It makes everyone around you feel better.
- *Teach your children to be happy about themselves* and to concentrate on inner qualities, confidence, and intelligence rather than weight, breast size, or physical characteristics.
- *Encourage your children* to work beyond the "perfect" expectations. "Perfection" does not exist.
- *Guide your children's food choices* instead of choosing for them. Having a wide variety of food choices in the house will allow your family to learn to select healthy food options.
- *Focus on health and behaviors that will foster healthy lifestyle habits.* Eat together as a family, discourage watching TV while eating, involve the children in shopping and meal preparation, encourage slower eating, do not overly restrict sweets, and do not use food as a reward or punishment.
- *Offer to make an appointment with a dietitian* for a healthy meal plan.
- *Try not to make an overweight child feel like the odd person out.* Prepare healthy meals and provide healthy snacks the entire family is expected to eat.

Here are some simple alternatives that will encourage healthier eating for the entire family:

Popular Choice	Healthier Choice
Breakfast:	
doughnuts, French toast, eggs, and/or bacon	whole grain cereal with low-fat milk, egg white omelet with Canadian

Popular Choice	Healthier Choice
	bacon, and fresh fruit or 100% juice
Lunch:	
cheeseburger, hot dog, pizza, or cheese sandwiches	low-fat lunchmeats (turkey, lean roast beef, ham), cheese, or low-fat peanut butter sandwiches
French fries or potato chips	pretzels, baked chips, or crackers
mayonnaise	low-fat mayonnaise, mustard, or plain yogurt
cola drinks	water, low-fat milk, 100% fruit juice
Dinner:	
steak, burgers, pizza, or fried chicken	lean or extra lean beef, pork, lamb, fish, skinless chicken, or turkey
French fries, cheesy potatoes, fried rice, or pasta with cream sauce	baked or boiled potatoes, brown rice, rice pilaf, or pasta with marinara sauce
vegetables with cheese sauce or fried/tempura vegetables	steamed, boiled, or stir-fried vegetables
cola drinks	water, low-fat milk, 100% fruit juice
Snacks and desserts:	
ice cream or ice cream shakes	sherbet, low-fat frozen yogurt, or low- or nonfat ice cream
cake or cookies	angel food cake, graham crackers, or low-fat cookies or cake
chips or buttered popcorn	air-popped popcorn, baked chips, pretzels, or breadsticks
candy	fruits or vegetables with low-fat dip
pizza	homemade, low-fat pizza

Debunking Weight Loss Myths

We all know that adults look for gimmicks and quick fixes when it comes to dieting to lose weight. This holds true for our preteens and teens too. Let's discuss some of the more common myths.

Myth #1: "I just need to find the right diet to lose weight."
Many dieters claim they just have not found the right diet plan for them. They want one that includes the foods they prefer (whether balanced or not), is easy to follow, and provides quick results. If they could just find this "perfect" diet, they would lose weight and keep it off.

Research says otherwise. Studies show that most dieters gain back the lost weight within five years; only 5 to 10 percent keep the weight off. Unless a person is willing to change lifestyle habits, weight will not stay off.

Myth #2: "If a little weight loss is good, lots of weight loss is better."
It's correct to say that being obese can increase one's health risks. However, being too skinny does not mean a longer, healthier life. In fact, being too thin can lead to health problems like amenorrhea, osteoporosis, or being unable to rely on fat stores in times of sickness.

Myth #3: "I have to follow a diet forever, or I'll just regain what I lost."
It's true that eating healthfully will help maintain one's weight. However, as many experts have shown, diets do not work. Being on a restrictive diet can lead to cravings and emotional swings. Imagining you will restrict yourself to a limited eating plan for the rest of your life is setting yourself up for failure from the start. By including a balanced variety of foods from all food groups (including sweets in moderation), you can be comfortable with eating and maintain a healthy weight.

Myth #4: "The faster I lose, the sooner I'll reach my goal weight."
Actually, the opposite is usually true. People who lose more than one to two pounds per week generally regain their weight more often and more quickly than people who lose at a slower rate.

When food intake is restricted too severely, the body's metabolism adjusts to this change. The body does not burn calories as efficiently, as it tries to conserve its energy (calories). Basically, it holds onto the weight. Slow and steady wins the weight loss game.

FOODNOTE
Lose weight at a slow and steady pace to win the weight loss battle.

Myth #5: "Everyone else is on this diet, so if it works for them, I should try it too."

A great number of people we know are on a diet of some kind. But, if diets worked, then why do so many people have to return time and again to weight loss programs, and keep trying all sorts of diets?

The fact is that most people regain the weight they lose because *they do not learn how to eat healthily and maintain healthy lifestyle habits.* Most weight loss programs thrive on this fact. It keeps them in business.

Myth #6: "Bread is fattening."

As low-carbohydrate, high-protein diets gained popularity in the 1990s, bread and other complex carbohydrates got a bad name. The fact remains that bread and carbohydrates in general are major sources of energy and fiber in our diets. Gram for gram, carbohydrates have less than half the calories of fat. Basically, bread and complex carbohydrates are wise choices in a healthy diet. (But like anything else, bread can become fattening if eaten in excess.)

Myth #7: "As long as I only eat fat-free foods, I can eat as much as I want to."

This is probably the biggest mistake you can make in trying to lose weight. Calories *do* count. Fat-free foods still contain calories—often *more* than the original product because the fat calories have been replaced with sugar calories. The bottom line here is: *count all calories.*

Myth #8: "I'm just too busy to eat right."

Having a positive attitude and making healthy eating a priority is important if you want to control your weight. There are many healthy, convenient foods that can be eaten on the run. A little pre-planning in grocery shopping and meal preparation may be all that's needed.

FOODNOTE

People who tend to skip meals eat more calories overall because they tend to overeat when they are really hungry. Eating smaller meals throughout the day seems to keep hunger in control, allowing one to limit calories and use nutrients most efficiently.

Myth #9: "If I just stay away from fat, I'll be OK."

The truth is that Americans have become *fatter* since the introduction of the sugar and fat substitutes. When it comes to weight loss, it is important to eat small amounts of fat for nutrient needs as well as to provide satiety. People who avoid fat in their diet generally are not satisfied with their meals and are constantly looking for something to eat. This often leads to a greater caloric intake than if a little fat had been included in the first place.

FOODNOTE

"Low-fat" does not give you a license to overeat. A serving of lite, nondairy whipped topping has the same number of calories as the regular type. A serving of low-fat peanut butter has the same calories as the regular kind.

The Truth about Today's Weight Loss Strategies

To be healthy, it's important to eat and behave healthily. Learning to eat right by watching portions and including balance and variety in your meal plan may not be exciting, but that's what works. Forget about the gimmicky diets, products, and programs; it's important for parents to teach themselves and their families to eat healthily and be healthy by getting back to the basics. And here they are.

One pound of fat equals 3,500 calories. When a person eats an excess of 3,500 calories during any period of time, a pound will be gained. When a person burns off 3,500 calories, a pound will be lost. If you take the 3,500 calories and divide it by 7 days in a week, you get 500 calories a day that you would need to add or subtract from your normal intake to gain or lose a pound in a week. Therefore, if you need to eat 2,000 calories a day to maintain your current weight and you eat 2,500 calories every day for a week, you will gain a pound that week. If you eat 1,500 calories every day for the week, you will lose a pound.

Many fad diets make outrageous promises of three or more pounds of weight loss per week. This loss would not be all fat, but more likely a lot of water and, possibly, muscle. And when carried to an extreme, vital muscles, such as the heart and lungs, could be affected. Yes, you or your child might note a decrease in the number on the scale with these types of diets, but chances are this will be *temporary,* as water weight quickly returns. That is why people get discouraged with diets and go from one to the next. These types of diets are especially *not* recommended for children and teens, who are growing and trying to build and maintain muscles.

In order to diet properly, balanced diets need to be followed. By cutting back a little at a time, limiting fats and sugars, and reducing portion sizes, calories can be decreased, and weight can be controlled. These small changes add up over time and help a person lose fat, not muscle or water.

When maintaining weight, a person must balance calorie intake with calorie expenditure.

To gain weight, a calorie increase needs to be achieved, where the calories consumed are greater than the calories burned.

To lose weight, the amount of calories burned off needs to exceed the calories consumed.

Weight loss is made possible by:

- lowering calorie intake
- increasing physical activity
- a combination of both

Yes, there are a number of diets people choose to follow that are nutritionally sound and lower caloric intake; but then again, there are many that can be harmful, especially to our youth. How can you tell if a diet is healthy?

An unhealthy diet plan:

- promotes quick weight loss (more than 2 pounds per week)
- encourages avoidance of one or more food groups
- encourages eating specific foods together, apart, or at certain times
- often uses celebrities to promote results
- promotes nutritional supplements that can be very expensive

- cannot be followed for long periods of time
- is not respected by health professionals
- does not give guidelines for maintenance, once desired weight is achieved
- uses words like "painless," "miracle results," "no-fail," and "cure-all" to describe it
- Promotes the program with descriptions such as "breakthrough program," "balances hormones," "enzyme process," and "secret formula"
- Includes the promise of "no exercise necessary" in its promotion

A healthy diet plan:

- encourages a lifestyle change that includes regular meals, snacks, and exercise
- encourages children to eat slowly
- allows foods from all the major food groups in moderate amounts
- promotes families eating together
- can be followed for extended periods of time without health risks
- allows planned snacks that keep children satisfied between meals
- does not use food as a reward or punishment
- is respected by health professionals

FOODNOTE:

The weight loss and fitness industry is a multimillion dollar industry and is getting bigger every year.

So, let's weigh the facts about some popular types of weight loss diets:

POPULAR WEIGHT LOSS DIETS

Type of Diet	Pounds Lost/ Week	Pros	Cons
High protein-Low carbohydrate	3 or more	none	water and muscle loss; weight often regained; high in fat and cholesterol; deficient in nutrients; can cause headaches and dizziness; poor long-term compliance
Very low calorie	3 or more	none	water and muscle loss; weight often regained; deficient in nutrients; poor long-term compliance
Commercially advertised store-front programs	2 to 4	teaches portion control; usually provides nutrition consultation; may offer specific programs for teens and children	often requires special food; may require nutrient supplements
Specialized hospital program	1 to 3	caters to specific ages; offers motivational support	difficult to find; can be costly
High-carbohydrate	1 to 5	high in fiber; can be effective if calorie and protein intake are adequate	severely restricts protein and fat; requires vitamin and mineral supplements; difficult to maintain over the long term

Type of Diet	Pounds Lost/ Week	Pros	Cons
Formula/ liquid diet	3 or more	helpful if used to replace no more than one meal per day	too few calories; water and muscle loss; weight often regained; poor long-term compliance; often low in nutrients.
Balanced diet	1 to 2	encourages all food groups; provides variety; offers adequate calories	none

---

FOODNOTE

The most effective way to lose weight is to *make lifestyle changes.*

From this analysis, it is clear that fad diets are generally not nutritionally balanced. Often nutrients are missing because the intake of grains, fruits, and vegetables is minimal. Other fad diets promote high protein and fat, which promote high cholesterol and heart disease—*not* a healthy path for your child to take. A large amount of protein also puts stress on the kidneys. This is the exact opposite of what the American Heart Association and the American Cancer Society recommend to prevent heart disease and cancer.

Fad diets are *not* magic. The reason weight loss occurs is that fewer calories are being taken in than are burned off. Since people cannot stay on these diets for long periods of time, any weight that is lost is regained, and maybe more. This pattern is not good for anyone, especially for a growing child.

FOODNOTE

Weight loss does not equal health.

Making Sure Any Diet Your Child Uses Is Safe and Healthy

Weight loss is *not* an easy process. When children try to lose weight, it becomes even more complicated. Children and teens who want and/or need to control their weight are still maturing sexually and growing. If they go on a fad diet to lose weight quickly and in an unhealthy manner, they run the risk of stunting their growth, impairing their sexual maturity, creating health problems, and initiating an eating disorder.

Having a healthy attitude about food is the most important first step toward eating well. What's that healthy attitude? For one thing, *food is neither good nor bad*. Food is not a pacifier nor should it be used to provide comfort or stimulation. Food should be thought of as a substance needed to provide nourishment for our bodies to grow and mature and to enable us to be healthy. All food *in moderation* can be included in a healthy meal plan. Yet because there are many so-called nutrition experts in our society, many misconceptions have developed about what is healthy to eat and about the best way to go on a diet to lose weight.

So many preteens and teens are looking for a quick and easy way to lose weight because in America, thin is "in." Pressure from peers, parents, and society in general has encouraged this dieting mania. Health professionals report that one half to two thirds of all teen girls and about one fourth of teen boys describe themselves as being overweight, (an excess of body weight due to bone, fat, and muscle; see the Body Mass Index charts on pages 12–13) even though only a small percentage are actually obese (a 20% excess of body weight solely due to body fat). As a result, our children are looking for ways to take off weight, often ineffectively and with unsafe methods.

WHAT'S A PARENT TO DO?

There are so many fad diets, diet drugs, and fat and sugar substitutes available to our children today to help them lose weight, it's scary. Most of us adults cannot tell if a diet or diet drug is safe, so how can we expect our *kids* to make healthy decisions? *What's a parent to do?* Here is some helpful information to share with your children when deciding whether or not to try a product, program, or diet:

- *Look for a safe program.* If the plan promises "quick" or "easy" weight loss, stay clear! Slow and steady are the keys. Losing weight too quickly (more than 2 pounds per week) will most likely lead to muscle loss. This can be dangerous and, sometimes, life-threatening.

- *If the diet sounds too good to be true, it probably is.* Stay clear when you see or hear these words: "fast-working," "painless," "guaranteed," "miracle diet," "secret formula," "no-fail," "cure-all," "breakthrough program," "lose fat forever," "balances hormones," "enzyme process," "no exercise."

- *Be cautious of weight loss camps for preteens and teens that are not run by trained professionals.* Too often food and calories are severely restricted so that afterwards, the lost weight is frequently regained. Also, such camps can be costly.

- *Choose a meal plan that includes all food groups, a variety of foods, has three meals and two to three snacks daily, does not forbid sweets or fats, and includes foods your child enjoys.* Encourage regular exercise, too.

- *Recognize that to date, safe weight loss drugs for children and teens have not been developed.* Weight loss drugs should never be given to children or teens under any circumstances. The Food and Drug Administration has banned many nonprescription weight loss drugs that claim to melt away fat, and the Federal Trade Commission has sued many of the companies that promote these products because of false claims.

- *Avoid diuretics and laxatives.* The weight that is lost with these drugs is *water weight.* If used in excess, dehydration can occur. And the weight will return once the person is rehydrated. Vital nutrients are the only things lost with these products. They do *not* promote fat loss. Also, laxatives can become addictive, and can cause severe damage to the colon.

- *Realize that fat substitutes are new to the market and are being modified and improved constantly.* At this point, most appear safe if eaten *in moderation.* However, long-term side effects are not well documented. If there is a question regarding a certain substitute, contact your physician or dietitian to obtain the latest information.

- *The sugar substitutes available on the market today appear safe, if consumed in moderate amounts.*
- *Think!* If a product or diet that is being promoted is so great, then why are not all of the health professionals encouraging it?
- *Remember that the federal government does not test, check, or license most weight loss programs.* A company or person does not need to be certified to run a weight loss program or sell weight loss products.
- *Check the qualifications of an author or spokesperson before believing what they have written or said.* To date, there are no regulations or qualifications needed to write a book or sell products on nutrition or diets.

It's not always easy to control which fads your child opts to use or follow. The hardest concept to learn is what "moderation" means with respect to food and diet products. Key points to keep in mind are to be a role model yourself, have a wide variety of healthy foods available, encourage exercise and activity, and keep the doors of communication open to discuss the latest diet trend(s) and the possibility of speaking to a dietitian about what is best.

6

MY CHILD'S A BEANPOLE!

Understanding the Special Concerns of the Naturally Underweight Child

Our society is often so focused on the desire to lose weight that it's easy to overlook the kids who want to or need to gain weight, either because they need to "bulk up" for a certain sport or because they are naturally underweight and need to gain weight to be healthier. In fact, it is just as hard—maybe even *harder*—to gain weight as it is to lose weight for preteens and teens.

Generally, kids who have a hard time gaining adequate weight have fast metabolisms, are very muscular, and/or do not have the interest or time to eat enough to meet their weight gain needs. Genetics also play a part in weight gain. Sometimes the child just does not know how much or what to eat to gain adequately.

For someone who does not want to be skinny, having a low weight can lead to body image problems, just as being overweight can. This is especially true for boys, who prefer to have a muscular, macho look versus the scrawny, peewee look. Underweight girls, especially when they enter high school, do not want to look like they are still in junior high school. Yet their bodies will not mature unless they eat healthily.

FOODNOTE

Being underweight can be just as difficult for kids as being overweight.

It is often difficult to tell if your child is naturally thin or has an eating disorder. In general, your child probably does not have an eating disorder if he or she shows an interest in eating, seems to be eating decent amounts of food, does not struggle to eat enough, is not obsessed with what he or she is going to eat or just ate, does not play with or hide any food, and can eat in most settings. Nonetheless, it never hurts to take your child to a registered dietitian for an diet evaluation to see if he or she is eating adequately. And if you suspect your child has an eating disorder, also refer to chapter 8.

WHAT'S A PARENT TO DO?

- *Take your child to a dietitian* for a balanced, healthy meal plan.
- *Encourage your child to keep a record* to monitor what's been eaten and what needs to be eaten to meet the diet plan guides provided by the dietitian.
- *Support and guide your child* in the changes that need to be made, without dictating what needs to be eaten.
- *Allow fried and high-fat foods more often.*
- *Top a potato with sour cream, heart-healthy margarine, and/or cheese.*
- *Offer larger portions of meats and protein sources.*
- *Use 2% or whole milk instead of low-fat milk.*
- *Encourage healthy, higher-calorie snacks,* such as milkshakes, puddings made with whole milk, and cheese or peanut butter and crackers.
- *Offer cereals and breads with higher fat content,* such as granolas and croissants.
- *Provide high-calorie foods in small or normal amounts.* Preteens and teens who need to gain weight have two difficulties. First, their stomachs are small and can only hold small amounts of food at one time. Second, their busy schedules make it difficult to find enough time to eat meals and snacks that will promote weight gain. So emphasize the higher-calorie foods. Here are some examples:

> croissant—240 calories vs. English muffin—160 calories
> whole milk—150 calories vs. skim milk—90 calories
> potato chips—150 calories vs. pretzels—80 calories
> tuna salad—380 calories vs. turkey—60 calories

- *Avoid products on the market that promote weight gain.* They are costly, may not taste great to your child, and are often not very satisfying. Instead, choose products, such as instant breakfast mixes that can boost the nutritional and caloric values of your child's diet.
- *Choose calorie-dense snacks from groups in the Food Pyramid* (see chapter 2) instead of selecting "empty calorie" foods that contain mostly sugar and fat and little nutritional value.
- *Sometimes, exercise will need to be limited to allow your child to add weight more easily.* If a preteen or teen is constantly participating in physical activities, this will make it even harder to put on weight.

All in all, the healthiest way to encourage weight gain in a child or teen is to increase the amount of food in a well-balanced diet and offer calorie-dense snacks more frequently.

7

MY CHILD WON'T EAT
Handling the Picky Eater

When our children were small we dealt with common food jags—periods of time when they wanted the same foods over and over again. Sometimes we thought we'd never see the end of macaroni and cheese, pizza, peanut butter and jelly sandwiches, grilled cheese, chicken fingers, hamburgers, or bologna sandwiches. Yet, some of our kids are *still* going through this stage! What can we do about it? Should we worry?

Children often learn to express their independence through their food choices. Because eating is one of the few activities children can control, they often tend to use food to get their way, to express opinions and feelings, or just to make a statement. Children request—or demand!—the foods they want and often refuse to eat if other foods are presented to them. Mealtime often turns into a battle between parent and child and becomes a no-win situation. Parents do not want their kids to go hungry so they often give in, allowing their children to feel they have won and have gained control. As years progress, the situation can get out of hand, and parents become frustrated if they don't know when and how to control it.

Young children are funny about their foods. They turn away if something looks strange, smells different, or even if one food touches another on the plate. Parents needs to be tuned in to not only their children's nutrition requirements, but also to their food preferences. We want to please our children, but oftentimes we want them to eat what *we* eat—and not necessarily in a manner they prefer.

As parents, we may believe that a variety of food choices and home-cooked meals are a must. We may think that if we can't offer the best to our children, we are incompetent as parents. We may also think that our children will like whatever we like. Not so!

Many children (young and old) would eat the same foods for lunch and dinner each day and be perfectly content; it's the *adults* who get bored with the same old foods. In many cases, when children get hung up on food jags, the foods they opt for are not all that bad after all. In fact, many are perfectly nutritious. But because each of us needs a variety of nutrients and balanced food choices, even the most nutritious foods cannot supply everything we need. This means other foods need to be incorporated into meals to achieve this balance and assure proper nutrition. There are ways everyone can work together to make everybody happy.

WHAT'S PARENT TO DO?

- *Allow children to help plan menus.* Let them have two to three nights each week to select and/or prepare their meal preferences. The control this offers them can go a long way towards getting them to be more agreeable on those nights on which other foods are being prepared.
- *Round out meals of favorite foods with other selections from the Food Pyramid* (see chapter 2). Add fruits, vegetables, and dairy products to balance the meal, and ask your child to eat a bite or two of these in addition to the main entrées. For example, macaroni and cheese with a little steamed broccoli, fresh fruit salad, and a glass of milk offers an adequate balance and variety.
- *Evaluate a three-day intake to make sure your concerns are justified.* Jot down everything that you know your child has consumed, and anything they tell you about in response to your asking. You may be relatively surprised at what is really being eaten.
- *Add a once daily multivitamin supplement to ease your mind.* Although it doesn't compensate for a healthy diet, such a supplement will reassure you that your child is at least getting some of the vitamins and minerals he or she needs. Make sure you choose a supplement that contains no more than 100 percent of the RDA for a child of that age.
- *Don't use bribes or punishments because of what is or isn't eaten.* Doing so teaches children to eat for the wrong reasons, that is, eating to please mom and dad or to avoid getting pun-

ished instead of to nourish one's body, which can lead to future problems regarding foods, emotions, and eating behaviors.

- *Don't make an issue over foods.* The more you push, the more your child will push you back.
- *Don't be a short-order cook.* Expect the entire family to eat what's prepared. If substitutes are allowed, your child won't be tempted to try new foods.
- *Don't assume that a food rejected before will never be accepted in the future.* Sometimes a child needs to see a food on the table a dozen times before actually feeling comfortable eating it.
- *Try the one-bite rule:* Encourage your child to try one bite, reinforcing that if he or she doesn't care for it, no more of it need be eaten. Doing this, however, introduces children to a wide variety of foods, and they may actually come to like a new food or two!
- *Remember that* everyone *has food preferences.* Be in tune to your child's favorites, and serve them with your favorites as well.
- *Set a good example.* If you don't sit at the table or actually eat certain foods, don't expect your child to either. Also, try to avoid the television and telephone during meal times. A parent who watches TV or talks on the phone during a meal will raise a child to do the same.
- *Be creative.* Try theme dinner nights (for example, Tex/Mex, Chinese, Italian, Halloween). Give your children a chance to offer suggestions, make placemats or napkin rings, set the table, or create special foods.
- *With older children,* discuss their health needs and how eating well benefits them.
- *Consider seeking professional help* for guidance and support, if necessary.
- *Invite a friend of your child's over to dinner* and find out, in advance, from the parent what some of that child's favorite foods are. If there's something new, or something that your picky eater doesn't usually eat—make it! Seeing a peer enjoy an unfamiliar or previously rejected food may make an impact on how your child feels about that food.
- *Keep in mind that children today are more food-savvy than they have ever been before.* By age six, children seem to know what

foods they like and where to get the foods they want. They learn from television, peers, and family members, and they want to speak their minds. Children know how to make many food decisions, are more brand-conscious, and want to have a say in what is bought and prepared. It's up to parents to take control. Give children a choice, *but* set appropriate limits.

Get Kids Involved in Food Preparation

Children who are involved in food decisions, food preparation, and meal setup are children who grow up with an appreciation of foods. They also take pride in their contributions and are better eaters overall.

When they are quite young, children should be allowed to help rather than be scooted out of the kitchen. Children who are encouraged to contribute at a young age will be more inclined to participate in years to come. Even a child as young as two years of age can help by putting bread in a breadbasket and napkins on a table. Older children can help prepare salads, mix batters, set tables, and even clean up. Weekly assignments should be made to all family members in order to teach responsibilities from a young age.

Children should also be encouraged to share their creativity in the kitchen. Just as youngsters enjoy building towers with blocks or playing with clay, cooking and baking in the kitchen offers them a creative outlet for their imagination. Don't worry about messes; messy kitchens can always be cleaned up. But seeing your children express their creativity and build their self-esteem is worth every mess they may make. Children as well as adults feel proud when they make something appealing and desirable. What a great way to build self-confidence!

Cookbooks and magazines offer many ideas to children of all ages. Bookstores, libraries, and even the Internet offer many resources for recipes and food ideas to keep fresh ideas coming into the kitchen. Teach your children to use these resources and offer assistance when they may need further guidance.

Children who learn their way around the kitchen at young ages grow up better prepared to manage responsibilities for feeding themselves and their families. They also are inclined to grow up with a greater love of *all* foods and cooking, along with understanding the benefits of good nutrition and its relationship to good health.

8

DOES MY CHILD HAVE
AN EATING DISORDER?
A Parent's Greatest Fear

Estimates indicate that there are more than eight million girls and women and one million males in the United States who suffer from eating disorders. It is estimated that between 5 and 20 percent will eventually die from their disorder. Experts do not know the cause of eating disorders, but they do know that most people with eating disorders have tried to lose weight by going on a diet. The following are common characteristics of people with eating disorders:

- They usually are intelligent and attractive.

- They have tried to lose weight by going on a diet.

- They are usually females between the ages of thirteen and twenty-two.

- They have gone through a major life change, such as a death in the family or of a pet, the onset of puberty, the birth of a sibling, or moving to a new town or a new school.

- They have undergone a trauma, such as sexual, verbal, or physical abuse.

- They are often athletes, especially involved in those sports that are affected by weight. Wrestlers, dancers, gymnasts, cheerleaders, and runners would be included in this group.

Eating disorders are more than just having problems with food. Generally, people who develop eating disorders feel a lack of control in their lives and use the eating disorder as a way to express a need. The decision to eat, starve, binge, or purge becomes a decision only they can control. When all other parts of their lives seem chaotic, developing an eating disorder gives them a sense of power and control. Unfortunately, the disorder eventually takes over all aspects of their lives: school, friends, family, hobbies, work, emotions, and health. They are consumed with thoughts of food, diet, and weight. These issues become such a priority in their lives that other life problems and situations are forgotten or avoided.

FOODNOTE

Eating disorders are not just about weight issues. They involve self-esteem, depression, power, and control issues, too.

It's important to recognize that more males are developing eating disorders than ever before (5 to 10 percent of people with anorexia or bulimia are males). In our society, boys or young men who cry or show their emotions are often looked down upon, so males learn to stifle their feelings. Boys are also pressured to be athletic, strong, and generally "macho." If these pressures are too great, an eating disorder can develop as an outlet for control.

Recognizing Eating Disorders in Your Children

According to dietetic professionals, *you should suspect an eating disorder if you have noticed that your child:*

- Often refuses to eat or eats very small amounts.
- Expresses an intense fear of becoming fat.
- Exercises to the point of exhaustion.
- Eats in secret or when others are not around.
- Disappears after eating or goes into the bathroom after meals.
- Experiences substantial changes in weight.

If you feel your child displays some of these behaviors, the best thing you can do is to bring your child to a doctor. Your physician can assess the situation further and make appropriate referrals, if necessary.

FOODNOTE

The person with an eating disorder is not the only family member who feels the pain.

The most common eating disorders are anorexia nervosa, bulimia nervosa, and compulsive overeating. A person can develop one or more of these disorders at the same time.

Anorexia nervosa, or anorexia, meaning loss of appetite, involves self-imposed starvation to maintain lower-than-normal weight. Anorexia affects one to three million Americans, mostly females in adolescence and early adulthood. Symptoms associated with anorexia nervosa include amenorrhea in women and failure to obtain menses in young girls; and a drop in hormone levels in boys and men. A loss of 20 percent or more of weight, weighing 85 percent of what is considered normal for height, or having a body mass index of less than 17.5 define anorexia nervosa. People with anorexia generally have a poor body image; they cannot visualize themselves as thin enough, and have an intense fear of becoming fat, which does not diminish as weight loss progresses. They consider food to be an enemy, even as they become progressively thinner.

FOODNOTE

Of young women who develop anorexia nervosa, 75 percent have had no history of being overweight.

Bulimia involves binge eating and purging. Bingeing involves stuffing oneself with tremendous amount of food in a short time. Purging is ridding oneself of the food either through vomiting, the use of laxatives and diuretics, and/or overexercising. Usually of normal weight, bulimics can more easily hide their disorder.

Once bingeing and purging become habitual, any stressful situation can trigger them to occur. A person may get temporary relief from performing these behaviors, but they are generally followed by tremendous feelings of depression and guilt. Bulimics have poor body image and try to please everyone. Unlike anorexics, who are pleased with their controlled starvation, bulimics are ashamed of their behavior(s). But, like anorexics, people with bulimia are obsessed with thinking about their weight and food.

Compulsive overeating, more common in males, involves uncontrolled episodes of eating, or eating large amounts of food on a regular basis, and is usually used as a way to combat stress and anxiety. Compulsive overeaters usually have a low self-esteem, eat very quickly and are usually not hungry when they eat. Junk food is usually the food of choice, and the food is eaten until the person is uncomfortably full. There is no purging in this disorder and large weight fluctuations are seen.

SYMPTOMS OF EATING DISORDERS IN CHILDREN

Anorexia

Changes in Body	Changes in Behavior
large weight loss in short period	strict obsessive dieting
loss of body hair	plays with foods/exercise
loss of menstrual period	obsesses with being/feeling fat
dry, yellowish skin	fears weight gain
extra sensitivity to cold	withdraws socially
frequent tiredness, but	refuses to eat anything with fat
difficulty sleeping	aims for perfection
abnormal bloating	
shortness of breath	
possible dental problems	
dizziness	
constipation	

Bulimia

Changes in Body	Changes in Behavior
weight loss fluctuations	makes frequent visits
dependency on diet pills,	to bathroom
laxatives, and/or diuretics	sneaks/hides food
severe dental problems	frequent bingeing
frequent sore throats	low self-esteem
loss of menstrual period	feels guilty about eating
sores or scars on back of hands	obsessively exercises
stomachaches or heartburn	feels depressed
puffy, swollen face	has mood swings
dehydration	

Compulsive Overeating	
Changes in Body	Changes in Behavior
excessive weight gain	finds comfort in food
tiredness/fatigue	consumes large amounts of
deterioration in overall health	food, especially in private
digestive problems	frequently diets
	has mood swings
	feels guilty about eating
	obsesses over calories
	and weight

The Side Effects of Eating Disorders

Anorexia, bulimia, and compulsive overeating have many side effects. If not treated, the end result can be death. Thus, it is extremely important to get medical and psychological treatment for someone with an eating disorder to prevent these complications, and to attempt to treat and ultimately cure the disorder.

Medical complications of anorexia include:

• Effects of starvation on the heart muscle may include low blood pressure, fainting, dizziness, and difficult breathing. Effects on the blood may include anemia, which leads to tiredness and weakness.

• Anorexics are at high risk for developing osteoporosis, a disease that causes weakening of the bones. This disease can start at any age, worsens as time goes on, and becomes quite debilitating. Osteoporosis is irreversible.

• Constipation and problems with the bowel are common. When the digestive system is not provided with enough food, it stops working correctly.

• Hormonal problems, especially in girls, are common. Young girls with anorexia often do not start getting their periods and girls and women who have begun menstruating often stop. During starvation, the body stops functioning properly. Adequate body fat, which is needed for normal hormonal production, is lost during starvation. This may permanently affect sexual development and maturation.

• Other side effects of anorexia include extreme cold sensitivity, insomnia, mood swings, growth of downy hair all over the body, and the loss of normal body hair.

Medical side effects of bulimia are:

• Dehydration occurs from purging due to laxatives, diuretics, and/or vomiting. If continued for a long time, an electrolyte imbalance can occur, causing kidney and heart complications.

• Anemia can occur, especially with laxative abuse.

• Dental complications from vomiting are frequent. Tooth discoloration and erosion from the gastric acid and vomited food are likely, in addition to mouth abscesses, blocked salivary glands, mouth sores, and bad breath.

• Other complications include damage to the tissue in the back of the throat or esophagus; stomach pain and ruptures; yellow-tinged skin; hair loss; and sores or scars on the back of the hand from sticking fingers in the mouth to induce vomiting.

FOODNOTE

A binge could consist of anywhere from 1,000 to 50,000 calories.

Medical complications of compulsive overeating include:

• The major side effect of eating in excess is obesity.

• Obesity and morbid obesity lead to heart disease, circulation problems, some cancers, and breathing problems. These diseases can begin at young ages.

WHAT'S A PARENT TO DO?

• *Identify which of the following statements pertain to your child.* The more items selected, the greater the likelihood that an eating disorder exists or is evolving. (Remember, however, that your child may not admit these behaviors to you. If you believe this is the case, a health professional may be able to assess the situation more accurately.) If one statement is relevant to your child, you may wish to keep an extra-cautious eye on his or her behavior. If two or more statements pertain, it is time to seek further advice from your child's doctor.

> *I spend most of my day thinking about what to eat or not to eat.*
> *I lie about what I eat.*
> *I like to cook, but I do not like to eat what I cook.*
> *I feel guilty when I eat.*
> *If I start eating normally, I won't be able to stop.*
> *I play with my food—cut my food into small pieces, push it around with the fork, hide it, and destroy its appearance.*
> *I don't like it when people watch me eat or eat with me.*
> (girls) *My menstrual cycles are irregular or have stopped.*
> (boys) *My sex drive is not present.*
> *I compensate for eating by exercising.*
> *I weigh myself more than once a day; the number on the scale upsets me.*
> *I have vomited or taken laxatives after eating so I won't gain weight.*
> *I feel fat, even though people tell me I'm thin.*

- *Objectively review your own relationship with food.* If you find yourself obsessing about dieting, fat grams, calories, and exercising, you may be sending negative messages and setting your child up for developing an eating disorder.
- *Confront your child in a supportive manner.* Discuss your concerns that he or she may have an eating disorder. Remember not to nag or yell.
- *Often the best way to start is by taking your child for a physical examination.* The doctor can rule out any physical problems and can support you in getting further help.
- *Educate yourself* and research treatment and support groups in your town.
- *Remember that eating disorders stem from complex problems relating not only to food, but to relationships with oneself and others.* Involving a therapist and dietitian who specialize in eating disorder treatment is a must. Note: A team approach by the professionals involved is encouraged.
- *As a parent, be supportive but not intrusive or overbearing.* This is sometimes difficult when you see your child behave in unhealthy ways. However, open lines of communication

and trust needs to be developed for a more successful recovery process.

- *Be persistent and consistent in getting your child the help that is needed*. Frequently, preteens and adolescents with eating disorders are resistant to treatment and therapy. They may try to hide their behaviors and symptoms to project the image that all is well. You need to show them that you are committed to helping them. This is probably the greatest responsibility you have as a parent.

Recognizing and then recovering from an eating disorder is a difficult process. Not everyone who goes for help succeeds, but it is important—indeed, critical—to put all efforts into helping your child recover from an eating disorder. The sooner you act, the greater the chance of recovery. Make your child's treatment process a priority in your life. However, even after treatment is completed, it is always wise for parents to be aware of possible reoccurrence. It may take years, and often a lifetime, to fight the lingering effects of eating disorders.

9

THE VEGETARIAN CHILD
Is My Child Getting the Right Nutrition?

Periods of preteen and teen years are defined by claiming independence, shaping personalities, and growing to maturation. It is also a time to share opinions and beliefs about social causes and life in general. Sometimes a child believes that eating food that comes from animals is inhuman, wrong, or even disgusting. Without any thought beyond saving the lives of animals, your child may proclaim an intention to become a vegetarian.

Adolescents are particularly drawn to vegetarian diets mainly because of their opposition to killing animals. Another reason for the decision comes from a belief that meat products are too high in fat. Since many teens want to be thin and stay thin, they think it is wise to avoid the fat found in meat products.

FOODNOTE

According to a survey reported by the Teenage Resource Group, 36 percent of teen girls—or twice as many as teen boys—consider it "in" to be a vegetarian.

Years ago, vegetarians were considered radicals. Now vegetarianism is a way of life, and many adults who are vegetarian are choosing to raise their children as vegetarians as well. Health benefits, such as reduced incidence of some cancers, obesity, heart disease, and chronic illnesses; along with cultural, social, and religious reasons, all contribute to choosing to follow this practice.

Some families, teens, and preteens choose to follow a nonmeat diet, yet do not consider themselves vegetarians. There are so many nonmeat food sources available today, it is possible to plan healthy, well-balanced meals without the inclusion of meat.

But just choosing to be a vegetarian does not make a healthy diet overnight. Meals and snacks need to be planned carefully to ensure proper nutrition. In fact, vegetarians often need to spend a little more time and thought on meal planning than other people do.

THE THREE MAIN TYPES OF VEGETARIAN DIETS

Type	What's Excluded	What's Included
lacto-ovo	meat, poultry, fish	eggs, dairy, fruits, vegetables, grains, seeds, legumes, nuts
lacto	eggs, meat, poultry, fish	dairy, fruits, vegetables, grains, seeds, legumes, nuts
vegan	all animal products (some vegans also exclude honey)	fruits, vegetables, grains, seeds, legumes, nuts

A Food Guide Pyramid has been developed for the lacto-ovo vegetarian and is illustrated on page 88. The recommended number of servings of grains, fruits, vegetables, and dairy products is identical to that recommended in the regular Food Guide Pyramid. The primary difference between the two is the exclusion of meat poultry, and fish in the vegetarian pyramid. Legumes, nuts, seeds, and eggs, along with the dairy products, provide primary sources of protein. For individuals following stricter forms of vegetarian diets, where eggs and dairy products may be avoided, special care must be taken to get the appropriate amounts of protein. (Note: It is important to keep in mind that most of us eat too much protein on a daily basis. Most teens and preteens only need between 40 and 60 grams of protein per day.)

Getting Enough Protein

If followed properly, a vegetarian diet can be healthy for all ages. Yet any meal or snack must include adequate protein, vitamins, and other important nutrients. When dairy products and eggs are a part of the

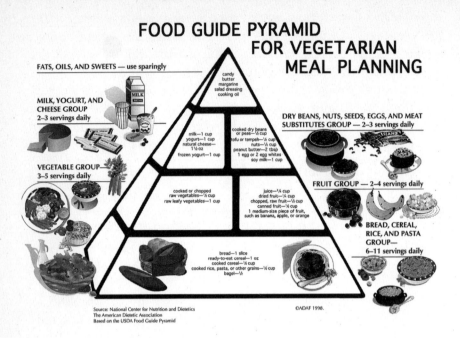

FOOD GUIDE PYRAMID FOR VEGETARIAN MEAL PLANNING

FATS, OILS, AND SWEETS — use sparingly

candy
butter
margarine
salad dressing
cooking oil

MILK, YOGURT, AND CHEESE GROUP
2–3 servings daily

milk—1 cup
yogurt—1 cup
natural cheese—
1½ oz
frozen yogurt—1 cup

DRY BEANS, NUTS, SEEDS, EGGS, AND MEAT SUBSTITUTES GROUP — 2–3 servings daily

cooked dry beans
or peas—½ cup
tofu or tempeh—½ cup
nuts—½ cup
peanut butter—2 tbsp
1 egg or 2 egg whites
soy milk—1 cup

VEGETABLE GROUP—
3–5 servings daily

cooked or chopped
raw vegetables—½ cup
raw leafy vegetables—1 cup

juice—¾ cup
dried fruit—¼ cup
chopped, raw fruit—½ cup
canned fruit—½ cup
1 medium-size piece of fruit,
such as banana, apple, or orange

FRUIT GROUP — 2–4 servings daily

BREAD, CEREAL, RICE, AND PASTA GROUP—
6–11 servings daily

bread—1 slice
ready-to-eat cereal—1 oz
cooked cereal—½ cup
cooked rice, pasta, or other grains—½ cup
bagel—½

Source: National Center for Nutrition and Dietetics
The American Dietetic Association
Based on the USDA Food Guide Pyramid

©ADAF 1998.

Food Guide Pyramid for Vegetarian Meal Planning

diet, it is not difficult to ensure complete sources of high-quality protein. Vegetarians can also get their protein by incorporating various types of soy in the diet. Soy products, which are abundantly available today, offer high-quality protein in many useful forms such as meat analogue products, tofu, tempeh, soy nuts, and soy milk.

The vegan diet, which includes only plant foods, requires more careful planning because most plants contain incomplete forms of protein. In order to make a complete protein from plants, a variety of plant foods needs to be eaten throughout the day. For example, grains combined with legumes give the benefit of bringing together various components of protein to make a complete source. The following chart shows what other foods can be combined to make a complete protein.

FOODNOTE

Parents need to ensure that their vegetarian child is getting enough protein and iron in their diet.

COMPLEMENTARY PROTEIN CHART

List 1	List 2
lentils	whole enriched grain breads
soy	whole enriched grain cereals
tofu	whole enriched grain pasta
nuts	corn
seeds	potatoes
tempeh	
peas	
dried beans	

NOTE: *Combine food(s) from list 1 with food(s) from list 2 to make a complete protein.*

Getting Adequate Nutrients

A nutrition concern for very strict vegans is possible deficiency of vitamin B_{12}. This vitamin, only found in animal products, may need to be supplemented into the diet at the advice of a physician. If dairy products are eliminated as well, inadequate levels of vitamin D may occur. However, the body is capable of producing enough vitamin D when it is exposed to the sun. Vegans who live in areas where there is no or little sunlight would be at risk for vitamin D deficiency and may need a supplement.

Other nutrients that should be carefully watched, and particularly so in vegan diets, include calcium, iron, riboflavin, and zinc. However, if managed properly by including a variety of foods in this limited diet, these nutrients can be adequately found in plant products.

Food Sources of Various Nutrients Useful to Vegetarians

- *Protein:* chickpeas (garbanzos); dried beans; lentils; soybeans; tofu; tempeh; rice, barley, and other grains; peanuts and peanut butter; milk, cottage cheese, yogurt, cheese; potatoes; pasta; bread

- *Calcium:* milk, cottage cheese, yogurt, cheese; soy milk; tofu; dark green leafy vegetables; dried figs; fortified orange juice; dried beans

- *Iron:* tofu and other soy products; whole grain breads and cereals; wheat germ, nuts and seeds; dried beans, lentils, garbanzo beans, split peas; dried fruits; prune juice; dark green leafy vegetables; watermelon

- *Riboflavin:* milk and dairy products; eggs; dark green leafy vegetables; legumes; enriched breads and cereals

- *Vitamin B_{12}:* milk, cottage cheese, yogurt, cheese; eggs; soy milk, soy burgers; fortified cereals

- *Zinc:* milk, cottage cheese, yogurt, cheese; eggs; dried beans, lentils, split peas; wheat germ, whole grains; seeds, nuts, peanut butter

When these foods are excluded in a particular meal:	Add these foods:	To get these nutrients:
meat	milk, dairy, grains, legumes, soy products	protein, iron, vitamins
poultry	legumes, soy foods, dark green vegetables	protein, riboflavin, vitamins
grains products	legumes, dairy	protein, iron, calcium, zinc
legumes	whole grains, dairy foods, dark green vegetables, nuts, tofu, soy products	protein, iron, calcium, zinc

FOODNOTE

Family members may choose to eat different foods, but they can still eat at the same time, at the same table.

Debunking Common Vegetarian Myths

There are some common myths about being vegetarian and vegetarian diets. Let's clarify some of these misunderstandings.

Myth #1: Vegetarian diets are healthier.
Although vegetarians do not eat the extra saturated fat and cholesterol commonly found in animal products, their diets can still be high

in fat from products like margarine, cream, cheese, fried foods, dairy products, and eggs. Too many starches, such as potatoes, pasta, and bread, can also distort the overall diet as can snack foods such as French fries, cookies, pies, cakes, candy, and other sweets. It all takes careful planning. Any diet can be healthy if planned properly.

Myth #2: Vegetarians cannot get enough protein in their diets.

Too much emphasis has been placed on adequate protein in the diet. In fact, we need only a modest amount of protein for our body's requirement. Lacto-ovo and lacto vegetarians have an easier time getting protein as compared to vegans, but it is possible to eat adequately without too much difficulty. Because plant foods are known as "incomplete" protein sources (since they do not have all of the protein building blocks called *amino acids*), various types of foods must be combined in the diet to make complete sources of protein as we've just seen in the table presented earlier in the chapter. Beans combined with grains, peanut butter on bread, and rice with lentils are just a few examples of how these complete proteins can be formed.

Myth #3: Children should not follow a vegetarian diet.

People of *all* ages can eat healthily by following a vegetarian lifestyle. However, in both vegetarian and nonvegetarian diets meals and snacks do need to be carefully planned in order to obtain all necessary nutrients. Too many foods from one food group and too few from another can lead anyone in the wrong direction. Because children are growing and developing, they need to eat a variety of foods from all the different food groups. Refer to the Vegetarian Food Guide Pyramid earlier in this chapter for assistance.

Myth #4: Vegetarian diets are low in fat.

Vegetarian diets can be low in fat or they can contain a lot of fat; it all depends on what foods are chosen. For example, people who worry about getting too little protein may opt to eat too much cheese, especially higher-fat cheeses. Vegetables themselves are low in fat, but if too much margarine, butter, or sauces are added, the fat content can rise quickly. Olives, nuts, seeds, and avocados also are high in fat. It's all a matter of choosing foods within moderation and selecting lower fat varieties when available.

Myth #5: In order to get a complete protein, certain combinations of foods have to be eaten at the same time.

At one time, this was thought to be the case, but researchers have found that this is no longer true. Combining various plant foods does help ensure that a diet includes all the essential amino acids needed to make a complete protein. You do not have to combine these foods together at the same meal, but should incorporate a good combination over the course of the day. These foods can be eaten not only together, but within meals of each other, too.

Myth #6: Vegetarian diets are boring.

Any diet can be boring. It just takes planning to include new choices every day. Seeking new recipes and foods ideas can be fun regardless of what kind of diet a person is following.

The sample menus below illustrate vegetarian meals that are healthy and can be enjoyed by you as well as your child.

Lacto-Ovo Vegetarian	Lacto Vegetarian	Vegan Vegetarian
Breakfast		
hard-cooked egg, whole wheat toast, fortified orange juice	whole wheat pancakes, banana, low-fat milk	whole grain cereal with soy milk
Lunch		
split pea soup, toasted cheese sandwich, fruit cup	soy burger on whole grain bun, tossed salad, cantaloupe wedge	meatless chili with beans, whole wheat crackers, tossed salad with garbanzo beans and sunflower seeds
Dinner		
soy meatloaf, mashed potatoes, steamed broccoli, whole wheat roll, applesauce	whole grain pasta with vegetables and beans fresh pineapple	stir-fried tofu, vegetables, pasta, whole wheat roll, fruit salad
Snacks		
yogurt or vanilla wafers and low-fat milk	rice cakes and low-fat milk	peanut butter on graham crackers

Other ideas for vegetarian meals (which can be used even if you are not vegetarian!) are as follows:

Breakfast:

cooked oats with nuts and raisins

egg alternatives

French toast or pancakes with fruit spread

ready-to-eat cereal (hot or cold)

bagel or English muffin with vegetarian sausage patty

Lunch:

salad bar

vegetable, lentil, or bean soup

meatless pasta or stir-fry

peanut butter sandwiches with jelly, fruit spread, or applesauce

vegetarian pizza

Dinner:

pasta or bean salad

rice pilaf or risotto

vegetarian lasagna, chili, or pot pie

vegetarian tacos

tofu stir-fry

stuffed baked potato

WHAT'S A PARENT TO DO?

- *Support your child's food choices as long as they are balanced.*
- *Learn what you can about vegetarianism.* Seek information appropriate for teens from books, magazines, libraries, websites, organizations, and registered dietitians.

- *Prepare pasta and rice dishes with a variety of vegetables.*
- *Try vegetarian soy burgers,* soy ground "beef," soy "hot dogs," soy "lunchmeats," soy breakfast "meats."
- *Make soups* with beans, lentils, and dried peas.
- *Combine cooked dried beans, peas, and lentils with rice* for pilafs; add them to tomato sauce; or mash them into spreads for sandwiches or spreads.
- *Prepare dinner omelets* or fritatas filled with vegetables and cheese.
- *Try including nuts and seeds* in muffin and bread recipes, in salads, or in stir-fry meals.
- *Offer meatless chili* made with different types of beans.
- *Be adventurous with ethnic foods* that include many combinations of vegetables, beans, and more.
- *When eating out,* ask restaurant staff about the nonmeat options they may offer—yet be sure to watch the fat in all of the dishes you try. Even without meat, fat content can be high. Always opt for low-fat versions of dairy foods and convenience and prepackaged foods.

Cooking and eating vegetarian can be as easy or as complex as you want to make it. Parents should remember that it's important to keep an open mind and give it a try. If planned well with variety of food choices, a vegetarian diet can be healthy for you as well as your child.

10

WHAT IF MY CHILD HAS A FOOD ALLERGY OR SENSITIVITY?

Discussion about food allergies has become so common these days that many parents think their children are suffering from a food allergy if they scratch their skin too often, have too many stomachaches, or get a heat rash! Although some people—about 2 percent of adults and up to 8 percent of children—do have food allergies, many more parents and kids have *food intolerances,* which differ from true food allergies.

A true *food allergy* occurs when the body recognizes that a food or substance eaten is foreign to its system and, in return, produces an antibody to stop the "invasion." When this happens, symptoms occur in the body such as swelling, cramping, vomiting, diarrhea, hives, rashes, or breathing problems. A person who suffers an allergic reaction must then avoid the allergen or food substance entirely. Allergies in children most often center around cow's milk, eggs, wheat, tree nuts, peanuts, fish, shellfish, and soy. Many times, these allergies occur when the child's body is not yet mature enough to handle the substance. As time passes, many children outgrow their allergies.

FOODNOTE

The most common symptoms of food allergies include rashes, hives, eczema, vomiting, and diarrhea.

If your child is allergic or sensitive to these foods:	Be cautious of these foods:	Avoid products with these items:
milk	milk and dairy products, ice cream, puddings, yogurt, cheese, baked products, breads, salad dressings, frozen desserts, creamed foods and soups, and processed lunch meats. Check labels on diet drinks, gravy mixes, and egg substitutes.	casein, caseinate, casein hydrogenate, dried milk solids, lactolbumin, lactate solids, sweetened condensed milk, whey or whey solids
eggs	eggs, mayonnaise/ mayonnaise products, baked goods made with eggs, egg pasta, pancake mixes, breaded products and sauces, such as hollandaise or custard sauce	albumin, dried egg solids, globulin, ovomucin, ovomucoid, ovoglobulin, livetin, vitelin
soy	tofu, soy sauce, soy products, lecithin-containing products, modified food starch, and tempeh	hydrolyzed vegetable protein, soy concentrate, soy protein, soya flour, textured vegetable protein, vegetable protein concentrate

If your child is allergic or sensitive to these foods:	Be cautious of these foods:	Avoid products with these items:
shellfish	lobster, shrimp, clams, crab, scallop, mussels, and other shellfish	surimi (a fish product used to make imitation crab, lobster, and some processed meat
fish	salmon, tuna fish, swordfish, other types of seafood, and products made with fish stock	surimi
tree nuts	walnuts, almonds, cashews, pecans, pistachios, macadamia nuts, brazil nuts, chestnuts, mandelonas, hickory nuts, filberts, artificial nuts, caponata, almond paste, nut pieces, pesto, nut butters, pine nuts (pinyon and pignolia), marzipan; some ice cream, baked products, breads, cereals, and salads; prepared vegetarian, Chinese, Thai, African, Indonesian, Mexican, and Vietnamese dishes	gianduja (a nut mixture found in some chocolate), natural and artificial flavorings

If your child is allergic or sensitive to these foods:	Be cautious of these foods:	Avoid products with these items:
peanuts	peanut butter, peanut flour, cold pressed, expelled, or extruded peanut oil; Nu-Nuts flavored nuts, trail mixes, mandelonas, beer nuts, mixed nuts, monkey nuts, marzipan, sunflower seeds, tree nuts, nougat and caramel candies, nut meats; some chicken salads, egg rolls, and chilis; enchilada sauce; some breads, ice cream, cereals, baked goods, candy and salads; prepared vegetarian, Chinese, Thai, African, Indonesian, Mexican, and Vietnamese dishes	natural and artificial flavorings, arachis oil (another name for peanut oil)
wheat	crackers, cereal, white and wheat bread, bran muffins, pizza, pancakes, waffles, gravy mixes, luncheon meats, salad dressings, breaded products, and some alcoholic beverages	wheat germ, semolina, graham, bran, all-purpose flour, pastry flour, cake flour, gluten flour, farina, modified food starch, malt or cereal extract

Eating an allergic food or substance *can* cause extreme illness or even death in some people. As little as 1/5,000 of a teaspoon of the problem food has been known to cause death. *Anaphylaxis* is a rare, but often, fatal condition where several parts of the body experience severe allergic reactions: airways can close, breathing may become difficult, and blood pressure drops. If this occurs—and often it occurs rapidly—it is life-threatening and immediate medical attention is necessary. So, it is also important to seek out all food products that contain allergic food substances and work with your child to be sure he or she understands the problems associated with consuming these foods. There is no cure for food allergies other than strictly removing the food from the diet.

Food intolerances, on the other hand, result from the way an individual's body metabolizes the food or substance, rather than from a problem associated with the body's immune system. A typical example of food intolerance is difficulty digesting milk, called lactose intolerance. Some people may have difficulties digesting milk because their body is deficient in the enzyme lactase, which is needed to digest milk sugar (lactose). When milk is consumed, the affected person may get cramps and diarrhea. The severity of these cramps can intensify as the years progress. Lactose intolerance is particularly common in African Americans and those of Mediterranean and Hispanic descent. Persons affected with lactose intolerance must then find alternatives in their diet to manage the problem.

People with food intolerances can sometimes eat the problem food and have no symptoms whatsoever. At other times eating a very small amount may cause problems. Every case and every individual is different.

It is not unusual for some individuals to be sensitive to various food additives as well, such as the sugar substitute aspartame, the flavor-enhancer monosodium glutamate (MSG), and sulfur-based preservatives and food colorings. Individuals who are sensitive to these substances should avoid them in their diet. The FDA requires that food products containing these substances be labeled as such to allow consumers to make educated decisions about the foods they buy and eat. MSG, a common ingredient in Chinese cuisine, is also used widely in restaurants. Sensitive customers should always ask their servers to have their foods prepared without its use.

Whether your child suffers from a food allergy or intolerance, it is important to be evaluated by a physician. *Never* try to diagnose the problem yourself.

WHAT'S A PARENT TO DO?

- *If you suspect a food allergy or intolerance in your child,* visit your doctor for a full evaluation. If necessary, you will be referred to an allergy/immunology specialist.

- *Keep a diet diary.* Write down everything your child has had to eat and drink for one to two weeks. Log any symptoms, conditions or reactions you may notice and the time it took for these to appear.
- *Learn to read food labels.* You may be surprised to learn what food items are found in various products.
- *Always ask questions when eating out.* Find out how food is prepared and what ingredients are put in various dishes.
- *Seek assistance from food allergy support groups.* Recipes, helpful hints on reading food labels, and advice from other parents can be very beneficial.
- *Make sure your child knows what to watch out for* and what kinds of food can contain allergic ingredients, because you can't be with your child all the time and monitor everything he or she eats.
- *Inform school officials and parents* of your child's friends of the problem and of what to do if your child suffers an allergic reaction in their presence.
- *Bring new foods into your child's diet* and don't let your child eat more than he or she can tolerate.
- *If your child suffers from immediate food allergy symptoms, remove the food from the diet.* If symptoms develop slowly, and it is difficult to pinpoint the offending food, bring new foods into the diet and rotate foods in the diet as well.
- *Talk to your doctor* about whether your child should carry an EpiPen—an epinephrine auto-injector for emergency allergic reactions.

Remember, if you suspect your child has a food allergy or sensitivity, it is important to discuss this issue with your physician. Parents of food-sensitive and allergic children generally become the best label readers and most informative sources regarding food products.

11

MY CHILD, THE ATHLETE

It is often difficult for parents to know what diet information to believe, especially when it comes to diet and exercise. Questions of interest to parents of athletes include: How should the diet vary before and after competition? Are supplements needed, and are they safe? What is the best fluid replacement for kids? So let's discuss these issues.

Young people involved in sports need to eat healthily. Generally, an active child or teen can follow the same healthy meal plan that an inactive child follows, although often eating larger portions of most food groups.

To determine if your child is getting adequate nutrition, a food record can be kept by you or your child, and then analyzed by a registered dietitian. The reactions to their foods need to be recorded as well. For example, a young athlete needs to know if stomachaches occur after eating ice cream, or if dizziness occurs when breakfast is missed. The dietitian can formulate a food plan specifically for your young athlete based on the information given.

FOODNOTE

Whether training for competitive sports, working out for good health, or just having fun, what your child eats and drinks and when are the keys to athletic success.

Making Sure Your Athletic Child Is Getting Enough Nutrition

By monitoring height and weight, you can identify if a child's growth is adequate. Chances are good that if growth is good, then the nutritional intake is also good. Also, if there are minimal complaints of being tired and if your child is in good health and does not get sick easily, then your child is probably in good shape, nutritionally.

Let's review some of the major nutrients we all need. Active children and teens may need some extra portions of food to obtain these nutrients. On the other hand, their intake may be sufficient, as most children get more than what's generally needed.

Carbohydrates: The Energizers

There are two types of carbohydrates, simple and complex. Both provide us with energy. *Simple carbohydrates* come from sugary foods like candy and cookies, but are also in fruits and milk. They are quick sources of energy as they are digested and absorbed easily. *Complex carbohydrates* come from starchy foods and are digested much slower. They are found in breads, cereals, rice, and pasta. At least 50 percent of our calories, especially for the young athlete, need to come from carbohydrates, or "carbs," as they are commonly known.

Carbs, especially the complex type, would be the best source of extra calories for young athletes. Complex carbohydrates are generally good sources of many vitamins and minerals, as well as fiber, making them a healthy source of energy. Sugary sources of carbohydrates basically supply calories and energy without much nutrition attached.

Protein: The Muscle Builder

The role of protein in athletic performance has attained mythic levels and needs to be clarified. Young athletes need to eat protein in a balanced diet, but in *moderation*. Protein has no magical power with regard to performance or muscle building.

Because North Americans generally eat more than enough protein in their diets, they rarely require protein supplements. The athlete needs protein mainly for building muscles, healing injuries, and for growth and development. Yet eating larger-than-necessary amounts of protein does not improve the body's ability to perform these functions. In fact, protein in excess of an athlete's needs does not build bigger or more muscles. Larger-than-needed amounts of protein will be converted to fat in the body, and increase the risk of dehydration, as the kidneys have to work overtime to rid the body of excess residue from the protein. Therefore, more is not better, and can actually be more harmful than beneficial.

How much protein do athletes between eight and eighteen need? Usually, between .6 to .9 grams of protein per pound of body weight. This translates into approximately 40 to 60 grams of protein a day for most preteen and teen athletes. This amount can be met by following the Food Guide Pyramid (see chapter 2) and including an extra glass of low-fat milk or an extra serving (3 to 4 ounces) of meat during the day.

Remember, the main sources of protein in the diet are the meat group, the dairy group, and the grain group. The healthiest sources are low-fat animal and dairy or plant-based products.

Fat: The Concentrated Energy Source

Because Americans have eaten too much fat in their diets in the past, fat has gotten a bad reputation. But fat is an essential nutrient; the body needs it to function properly and healthily. Besides being an energy source and making our food taste good, fat helps the body absorb and transport the essential vitamins A, D, E, and K. It also supplies essential fatty acids to the body.

How much fat does a young athlete need? Fat needs to be used sparingly and wisely in the youth's diet. *No more than 30 percent of the total calories in a preteen or teen's diet needs to come from fat.* Also, it is best if the fat eaten is of vegetable origin. Low-fat animal products are also okay, if eaten in moderation. Lean beef and poultry without the skin are great sources of iron, minerals, and protein so important for the competitive athlete. Salmon and certain other fish are also good choices and offer heart-healthy benefits.

It is important not to severely restrict a child fat intake, as moderate amounts of fat are part of a healthy diet. However, if excess calories are being eaten in the form of frequent fried foods, desserts, snack foods, or fast foods, then the athlete may be getting too much fat and limits will need to be established.

Vitamins and Minerals: The ABCs of Healthy Eating

Food sources should be the major source of vitamins and minerals for young athletes. The body best uses vitamins and minerals if obtained from food. Supplements may be needed only if the young athlete is eating less than 2,000 calories daily.

Certain vitamins, such as A, D, and E, can become toxic if taken in larger-than-needed amounts. Symptoms like fatigue, headaches, loss of appetite, and muscle weakness can occur as signs of excessive vitamin usage.

Athletic youths need to be concerned about having enough of two major minerals in their diet. Calcium and iron appear to be needed in larger-than-normal amounts in active children and teens.

Calcium is needed to build and maintain strong bones and teeth. Between the ages of twenty and thirty-five, bones reach their peak density. It is hoped that during this period the bones have collected enough calcium to prevent osteoporosis and maintain strong bone structure for a lifetime. The best time to build bones is between ages nine and eighteen. The more attention paid to increasing bone structure during this time, the better. If inadequate calcium is consumed during the growing years, the body has to take calcium from the bones to keep the necessary levels of blood calcium normal. This process can weaken the bones and is irreversible.

Poor calcium intake often occurs in our youth for a variety of reasons. Some teens believe that milk is fattening and that milk and dairy products are not needed after childhood. Many young people just do not like milk and dairy products, have milk and dairy allergies, or are lactose intolerant. Children eight to eighteen *need* between 800 and 1,200 milligrams of calcium daily. Their bodies do not care if they do not like milk, do not want milk, or cannot have milk. It is important to get enough calcium. Low-fat milk and dairy products, fortified food products, and dark green leafy vegetables are the best sources of adequate calcium for preteen and teenage athletes. Supplemental sources of calcium may also be necessary at the recommendation of a physician or registered dietitian.

For competitive athletes, it is important to emphasize that calcium is needed for bone structure and strength and for muscle function. If injured, an athlete with adequate calcium stores will heal more quickly than an athlete who has not had enough calcium. Children with thin bones are more susceptible to stress fractures and other injuries.

FOODNOTE

Girls (and boys) who do not consume enough calcium may not reach their "peak bone mass," thus putting them at greater risk of osteoporosis in later life.

Iron is needed to carry the oxygen in blood. Yet athletes are more prone to iron deficiency anemia than nonathletes, as they lose more iron through sweat. Females lose even more iron through their menstruating. This makes teenage girl athletes at the highest risk for iron-deficiency anemia.

To make sure your child is getting enough iron, recognize that iron from animal sources seems to be better absorbed than iron from plant sources. Lean beef, poultry, and salmon are excellent iron sources. Plant sources include black, navy, kidney, and pinto beans; dried fruit; lentils; peanut butter; and spinach. Iron-fortified breads, cereals, and pastas are also good sources of iron and need to be eaten on a regular basis. Plant and grain sources of iron become especially important in a vegetarian diet. The body better absorbs iron from foods eaten in combination with a citrus food that contains vitamin C. Orange juice, kiwifruits, strawberries, and tomatoes are good examples of vitamin C-rich foods.

Water: Fill 'er Up

Water is probably the most important nutrient for the competing athlete. Kids generally do not drink enough water. They prefer soft drinks and flavored beverages. It is important for parents and coaches to encourage young athletes to drink water.

Compared with adults, preteens and teens need to drink water because:

- Children are more sensitive to temperature extremes.
- Children sweat less.
- Children have more skin area per body weight.
- Children get hotter during exercise.
- Children's hearts pump less blood than adult hearts.

For these reasons, children are more susceptible to dehydration than adults. Children have busy schedules and probably do not think about drinking water, so they must be reminded to drink water.

It is important to drink water before, during, and after exercise and competitions. *Heat illness is the most common sport injury that occurs today,* yet it is the most preventable. Dehydration can occur even with as little as 1 percent of body weight loss from fluid lost during an activity. That means just 1 pound lost in a 100-pound person! And if a child becomes dehydrated and unable to control his or her body temperature, endurance and performance will be diminished.

Here are some guidelines on how much your preteen or teen athlete should drink to prevent dehydration:

- *Before exercise:* one to two hours before the activity, a minimum of 2 cups of cool water—more if fluid loss is expected to be greater than normal

- *During exercise:* 5 to 7 ounces of cool water every fifteen minutes

- *After exercise:* 2 cups of cool water for every pound lost.

FOODNOTE

To test if you are adequately hydrated, check the color of your urine. A clear, almost colorless shade of yellow indicates good hydration.

Eating for Competition: Pre- and Post-Game Meals for the Athlete

What and when the young athlete eats on the day of competition is significant to the outcome of the competition. An upset stomach during the event can cause poor performance or even reason to drop out of the event. The pre-event meal needs to accomplish two tasks: 1) Prevent the athlete from becoming hungry during the event; and 2) Provide enough fuel to allow the athlete to compete efficiently.

The outcome of the athlete's performance will not only depend on his or her ability, but also on the nutrition practices of the week before the event as well as the pre-event meal. Variety and balance are key during the week prior to competition. Keeping convenience and fast foods to a minimum is also important. The pre-event meal should include complex carbohydrates and water. Large amounts of sweets and fats should be avoided, though moderate portions of protein and fiber are permitted.

Athletic youths should *not* eat simple carbohydrates before an event to give them an energy boost. The energy they will need to rely upon for the event will come from their food intake days and hours before actually competing. Here are two examples of healthy *pre-event* meals to be eaten three to four hours before the event:

Example 1

1 cup orange juice

1 slice wheat toast with jelly

a medium banana

1 cup low-fat yogurt

Example 2

small chicken breast

large baked potato with 1 teaspoon margarine

carrot sticks

1 cup low-fat milk

Examples of snacks to be eaten one to three hours before the event are:

bagel—plain; no cream cheese, butter, or margarine

bread—plain; no cream cheese, butter, or margarine

pretzels

fruit—choose low-fiber options such as plums, melons, cherries, peaches, or juice

After the competition is completed, it is very important to replenish the used energy stores and fluids. Fruit juice, a banana, a bagel, fruited yogurt, pretzels, and water are good suggestions. A meal should follow within five hours of the completion of the event, and it should consist of mainly complex carbohydrates. You can refer to the pre-event meal suggestions and add a little more fat and protein, or use the following postcompetition meal suggestions.

Example 1

spaghetti with meat sauce

fruit salad

Italian bread with olive oil

low-fat milk

Example 2

small chicken breast

large baked potato with 2 teaspoons margarine

green beans, dinner roll with 1 teaspoon margarine

low-fat milk

It may be easier for some children and teens to drink, rather than eat, right after the competition. Offer them 100 percent fruit juice or lemonade.

WHAT'S A PARENT TO DO?

- *Guide your athlete in proper nutrition.* If you are unsure of what to do, find a registered dietitian or book on sports nutrition.
- *Check with your young athlete* to make sure that enough fluid is consumed before, during, and after events.
- *Stay up-to-date* on the newest and most accurate information on nutritional needs for young athletes.

The most important job a parent has in feeding a young athlete is providing a healthy, varied selection of foods. Diets that are high in complex carbohydrates and fluids, moderate in protein, and low in fat will maximize the athlete's performance as well as provide for growth. It is also important to remember that a "kid is still a kid," so allow for an occasional treat, such as ice cream, candy, or chips. And don't forget to set a good example yourself and eat healthily.

12

HELP! MY CHILD ONLY EATS JUNK FOOD

Potato chips . . . soda pop . . . candy bars . . . cookies . . . doughnuts . . . chewing gum . . . presweetened cereals . . . cake . . .

Do these foods seem like staples in your child's diet? Many parents worry about their children's excess consumption of these types of foods and wonder whether there is any hope for a healthy lifestyle down the road.

Foods such as those listed above are often referred to as "empty-calorie foods." They contribute calories primarily from sugar and fat and offer little, if any, nutritional value. Too many of these types of foods in the diet can lead to poor health because they take the place of healthier food choices. Filling up on empty-calories foods leaves little room for the important foods needed by the body. Remember that empty-calorie foods or foods with higher sugar and fat content fall into the food group at the very tip of the Food Guide Pyramid (see chapter 2). This group should contribute the *least* amount to the overall diet.

Is Your Child Eating Too Much Sugar?

It has been reported that many people eat their weight in sugar each year. On average, this amounts to about 140 pounds of sugar per person per year. What does this say about our children? A regular 12-ounce canned soft drink alone contributes up to ten teaspoons of sugar! Drinking two soft drinks per day brings this up to twenty teaspoons of sugar. Would you knowingly give your child twenty teaspoons of sugar to eat? *Wow.* What an eye opener!

FOODNOTE

Soft drinks are the single largest source of sugar in the diet. Children currently drink twice as much soft drinks as they do milk.

Sources of Sugar	Serving Size	Amount of Sugar (teaspoons)
chocolate doughnut	1	4
ice cream	½ cup	4
iced cupcake	1	5
jelly	1 tbsp.	3
soft drink	12 oz.	10
hamburger bun	1	1
presweetened cereal	1 cup	3

FOODNOTE

To convert grams of sugar to teaspoons, divide grams by 4.

Look for hidden types of sugars, too, in the foods your child eats. All of the following are sugars:

honey	corn sweeteners
fructose	confectioners' sugar
molasses	dextrose
corn syrup	maltose
brown sugar	Mannitol
lactose	molasses
sucrose	Sorbitol
glucose	

When you see these ingredients on food labels, it means some form of sugar is in the product.

Sugar has often been blamed for hyperactivity in children. Yet the fact is that sugar acts more as a sedative than as a stimulant. To date, no scientific evidence has shown a connection between sugar and hyperactivity, but ongoing research continues.

Yes, our children are eating too much sugar, whether they are aware of it or not. The two major health risks of too much sugar are tooth decay and obesity. It is up to parents to set examples and provide moderate amounts of sweets combined with a balanced selection of other foods. Curbing the "sweet tooth" is necessary to improve the health of our children.

What About Fat?

We all hear about fat, read about it, and assume it's bad for us. But, as we know, our bodies still need some fat, albeit in small amounts. Still, health professionals urge people of all ages to lower their fat intake because major health problems, such as heart disease, obesity, and cancer, have been linked to excess fat.

The term "fats" encompass both saturated and unsaturated (polyunsaturated and monounsaturated) fats. *Saturated fats* are primarily found in foods that come from animals, such as milk, dairy products, meat, cheese, and ice cream, and in cakes, cookies, pastries, and other things made from butter and eggs. These fats can impact a child's cholesterol level, which can increase incidence of future health problems. *Unsaturated fats* are typically fats such as vegetable oils and those found in some seafood. These fats do not cause cholesterol levels to rise and do not lead to heart problems, but can still have an impact on weight gain if eaten in excess.

Current estimates are that most Americans eat upwards of 40 percent of their total daily calories from fat. Recommendations are to consume no more than 30 percent of total calories from fat sources, and some health experts believe this should be reduced to 20 to 25 percent.

Reducing intake of foods higher in fat and selecting leaner meat products, lower-fat cheese and dairy items, lower-fat dressings and condiments, and lower-fat snacks is key in reducing the total percentage of fat in one's diet.

But even foods that are too high in fat or sugar should never be forbidden for your child to eat. Banning a food just encourages children to want it more. Every food can be incorporated into a healthy diet—just plan healthier food choices around it! You should not rush to assume that your child is a poor eater overall just because she or he chooses one or two less nutritious food choices. It's the *overall* diet that needs to be evaluated, not just one or two foods.

Junk food diets can be modified to please everyone. Let's look at a typical junk food diet and simple alternatives that can be made to improve it.

Junk Food Diet	The Better Choice Alternative

Breakfast
 doughnut (1)   bagel (1)
 fruit drink   100% fruit juice
Lunch
 double cheeseburger deluxe   single hamburger with
 large French fries   lettuce/tomato
 16-ounce soft drink   small French fries
                                         2% milk

Snack
 potato chips   pretzels
 12-ounce soft drink   apple
Dinner
 extra crispy fried chicken   baked chicken breast
   (2 pieces)   mashed potatoes with
 mashed potatoes with gravy   margarine
 biscuit with butter   steamed broccoli
 16-ounce soft drink   dinner roll with margarine
                                         cantaloupe wedge
                                         2% milk

Snack
 pepperoni pizza (2 wedges)   1 cup popcorn

Nutrition analysis
 Total Calories: 2,824   Total Calories: 1,886
 Total Fat Calories: 1,054   Total Fat Calories: 520
 Total Fat Grams: 117   Total Fat Grams: 58

You can see that just by making small changes you can make major changes in the overall diet.

Here are some additional healthy options to keep on hand for quick snacks:

  string cheese
  cheese wedges and crackers
  fresh vegetables and dip
  fresh fruits
  dried fruits

graham and cinnamon graham crackers
celery with peanut butter
vanilla wafers
fruit filled cookies
gingersnaps

FOODNOTE

There are no good foods or bad foods, only good and bad eating habits.

WHAT'S A PARENT TO DO?

- *Find alternatives to soft drinks* by offering low-fat milk and water with meals. Limit soft drinks between meals.
- *Cut back on sugar* in recipes by 2 tablespoons to $\frac{1}{4}$ cup.
- *Add vanilla extract for extra flavor* in drinks and shakes.
- *Use canned fruits packed in fruit juice* rather than those packed in syrup.
- *Choose sugarless gum.*
- *Limit presweetened cereals.* Mix presweetened cereals with unsweetened ones.
- *Put sugar in a shaker* instead of a sugar bowl.
- *Limit juice,* even 100% fruit juice, to 4 to 6 ounces daily.
- *Limit fried foods.* Instead bake, broil, or steam.
- *Switch to low-fat dairy products.*
- *Switch to lower-fat salad dressings and mayonnaise.*
- *Try herbs and other seasonings* instead of butter and margarine.
- *Use lean cuts* of meats, skinless chicken, and fish.
- *Once or twice a week, try a vegetarian meal* with beans and tofu instead of meat.
- *Reduce intake of processed meats* like bacon; bologna, salami, and other cold cuts; hot dogs, pepperoni, and other sausages.
- *Use egg substitutes or egg whites* in place of egg yolks or whole eggs.
- *Limit convenience foods and snacks that have excess fat.* Pretzels and popcorn are a wiser choice than potato chips, and baked chips are a better choice than fried ones.

- *Reduce frequency of fast food dining* to no more than three times per week.
- *Read labels.* There is no better consumer than one who is informed.

Getting your children to minimize the amount of junk food eaten is not an easy task. You want your children to make healthy choices not only when they are with you, but also when they are with their peers, away from your watchful eye. It's important to educate them about why it's important to eat healthily, which includes eating *moderate* amounts of the more sugary and fatty foods along with fruits and vegetables and whole grains. By setting an example, providing a wide variety of healthy choices, and involving your children in food and menu selections, you also help establish good eating habits that hopefully will last through the teen years and into adulthood.

PART THREE

IMPLEMENTING YOUR FOOD SMARTS

13

BEING A GOOD ROLE MODEL

There is no better way to begin to implement your food smarts than to set a good example yourself. Telling children and teens to eat right just doesn't cut it; *showing* them is better. What parents teach from a young age . . . what parents bring into the home to eat . . . what parents do themselves . . . what parents eat themselves: *this* is how children learn.

Have you ever wondered how your eight-year-old son learned about reading food labels, or where your eleven-year-old daughter got the phrase, "I feel fat today," or why your fifteen-year-old feels he doesn't need to eat breakfast anymore? Look at yourself. Think back to what *you* do on a regular basis. You may see many of your old habits now reflected in your children. You may not realize the impact you have had on your children, but they have a keen sense for knowing what goes on around them. They pick up comments, habits, clues, and gestures so easily from the people they live with.

For example, various cultures eat certain types of traditional foods, especially for holidays and special occasions. How do you think your children develop a sense of taste and desire for these foods? Having a variety of foods available for your family to try time and again allows new foods to be accepted with greater success.

If you start right from the beginning of a child's life and create good habits at home, your children will learn to follow your example. Otherwise you may find your son wanting to eat dinner while he watches television or your daughter eating over the stove rather than at the table. Again, what have your children watched you do? Did you frequently catch your favorite TV program or grab a quick dinner while standing over the stove yourself? You may not realize the effect these habits have on your children, but even very young children are a lot smarter and more easily influenced than we may realize.

Besides, hasn't there ever been a time when you've acknowledged to yourself, "I've become my mother; I'm doing things exactly the way she did!"

Yes, it's difficult to change habits once they are developed and practiced for days, months, and years at a time. That's why it's always better to develop good habits from the start. But change *is* possible.

FOODNOTE

One good habit feeds another.

WHAT'S A PARENT TO DO?

- *Be a good role model.*
- *Know the importance of a healthy diet;* choose foods lower in fat and higher in nutrients.
- *Follow the Food Guide Pyramid* (see chapter 2); it helps you shop, plan, and eat better all around.
- *Teach cooking skills;* children who learn basic food preparation skills have a greater appreciation and understanding of foods. Kids who enjoy cooking are generally better eaters.
- *Plan family meals;* get everyone involved in planning, cooking, serving, and cleaning up. Families who eat together are often closer and communicate more effectively than those who do not.
- *Provide a variety of foods* and give your child the responsibility to select from those offered.

Getting Started on the Right Path

Food is a big part of life. Not only is it our fuel for living and surviving, but it's often the center of our social existence.

References to food are everywhere: We see food on television, read about food in newspapers and magazines, and can buy food on every corner in town. Somewhere within all this access to food we've forgotten its main purpose: to keep us *healthy* and alive. We need to constantly remind ourselves why we eat and learn to understand the relationship between food and health. Here are two things you should be sure to do.

1.   Begin with Breakfast

The word *breakfast* means to "break the fast." It's time to eat again after the body has fasted during the night. The body now needs to start its engine again, and get on with the day. It needs refueling to help stay alert, active, and focused.

Eating breakfast is a prime example of how, as a parent, you can influence your child's food behavior. Adults who rarely or never eat breakfast don't see this as being an important meal for their children. And while young kids may be more inclined to eat breakfast each morning as they are told, older kids tend to develop habits that mimic their parents' actions. In a family that sits down together each morning, even for only five or ten minutes, the children tend to form habits that they continue with, even when they become parents themselves. Yes, busy families often have different schedules at breakfast time, but if arrangements are made to create a breakfast schedule that meets the family's needs—or at least have some of the family to eat together— children will be more apt to build this habit into their lifestyles.

FOODNOTE

Students who eat breakfast actually score higher on tests and perform better in school than students who do not.

Time crunches, working moms and dads, and stressful mornings have moved us from a time of sit-down breakfasts of piping-hot pancakes, eggs, and toast to a life of breakfast treats and bars, or coffee shops. Yet grabbing a quick breakfast on the run and moving out the door should not take precedence over the importance of eating something to nourish and fuel our bodies for health.

Here are several breakfast energizers that might work for you:

fortified cereals with low-fat milk
yogurt with banana or strawberry slices

pancakes and waffles with blueberries
instant oatmeal with orange juice
hard-cooked egg, toast, and fruit spread
fruit-filled breakfast bar with low-fat milk
English muffin with peanut butter
rice cake with low-fat cottage cheese

WHAT'S A PARENT TO DO?

- *Try to plan breakfast to include a fresh fruit or juice,* complex carbohydrate, and low-fat milk.
- *Aim for a ten-minute weekday and fifteen-minute weekend breakfast with the family.*
- *Stock up the pantry, refrigerator, and freezer with quick, healthy options* including waffles, pancakes, bagels, fruit, instant oatmeal, and dry cereals.
- *Prepare larger breakfast portions of things like muffins and hard-boiled eggs on the weekend,* so you'll have leftovers for the weekdays.
- *Pack a bag breakfast for mornings on the go;* you might include dried fruit, 100% fruit juice boxes, bagels, muffins, cheese cubes.
- *Make cereal combinations.* Mix several kinds together for a fun cereal trail mix.

---

2. Aim for 5 A Day

Following the recommendation of five servings of fruits and vegetables is another example of how we can be good role models to our kids. You may think this habit is a bit hard to get your children to follow, particularly if you aren't a big fruit and vegetable eater yourself. Some days may go by when you wonder if your child ate any fruits or vegetables at all! As a parent, it is important to be aware of your child's diet and encourage more of these types of foods. Fruits and vegetables are very high in vitamins, minerals, and fiber; low in calories and fat; and make an excellent addition to meals and snacks throughout the day.

Debunking Myths about Fruits and Vegetables

Myth #1: Fruits and vegetables cost too much.

Fruits and vegetables are actually no more expensive than a typical pack of cookies. It's just that you notice the price more because prices of produce fluctuate with the seasons. If this becomes a problem for you, stick with seasonal choices and buy store specials. Or better yet, always keep canned and frozen varieties on hand.

Myth #2: Preparing fruits and vegetables is too much trouble.

Buy ready-to-serve products, like premade salads and baby carrots, or make a family project out of preparing the food. How much fun it would be to offer a family salad bar!

Myth #3: Produce is highly perishable.

"It just doesn't last in our house." Buy produce that is not totally ripe and be sure to keep it in sight. If you put a bowl of fresh fruit on the kitchen table, it's more apt to be eaten. If you hide it in the back of the refrigerator or in a drawer, it will never be used. Also, when fruits begin to get too ripe, peel them and freeze them or cook them. Make a compote or applesauce, for example. They can be used for fruit breads and smoothies.

Myth #4: Fruits and vegetables contain harmful pesticides.

Pesticides are actually used to help us, not harm us. They keep insects and diseases away from crops and ensure a more plentiful supply of fresh products. Pesticides used are highly monitored, tested, and regulated to make sure our food is kept safe. For those parents who may be especially concerned about pesticides, organic foods may be an option.

WHAT'S A PARENT TO DO?

- *Take your children to the grocery store.* Ask them to select two vegetables and two fruits they would like each week.
- *Set out a fresh fruit bowl each day and vary the selections.* When fruit is visible, it is often eaten more frequently. Snacking on fruit then becomes easier.
- *Try vegetables with dip before the dinner hour.* You can satisfy the late afternoon munchies and fill a vegetable requirement as well.

- *Take cut-up fruit, dried fruits, and vegetable sticks on car rides.* When there are no other snacks available, these foods become more appealing.
- *Serve and drink 100% fruit juices* instead of soda for an extra boost of nutrients.
- *Add fruit* to yogurt and cereal for breakfast.
- *Grab a banana* mid-morning.
- *Eat some grapes* after school.
- *Top baked potatoes or pizzas with steamed vegetables.*
- *Serve vegetable omelets.*
- *Add sliced tomatoes* to grilled cheese sandwiches.
- *Serve fruit kabobs* with meals.
- *Make muffins* with chopped fruits.
- *Try banana pancakes.*
- *Pack small boxes of raisins* in backpacks.
- *Add crunch to your child's lunch* with fresh carrot, celery, or pepper sticks.
- *Add frozen veggies* to pasta sauces.
- *Make a chopped vegetable salad buffet* for dinner.
- *Top frozen yogurt* with berries.
- *Make a smoothie* with low-fat milk or yogurt and frozen fruits.
- *Try mashed banana or applesauce* with peanut butter for a change.
- *Jazz up a dessert* with fresh fruit topping.

You never realize how your habits are passed onto your kids until you start to see your habits reflected in your children's behaviors. They can adopt either your positive or negative habits. Because of this, it is so important to model good lifestyle habits when your children are young, before unhealthy habits become the norm in everyday life.

14

PLAN YOUR MEALS, PLAN YOUR SNACKS

You can also serve as a good role model during other times of the day besides breakfast. Think about how you snack, how you cook, how much you eat, and how you exercise. All of these factors influence your child as well. Planning is the key to a healthy diet. No one can manage just to eat the right foods without some advanced planning. Whether seeking out recipes, writing a shopping list, preparing foods at home, or even having a dinner on the town, planning is necessary for all aspects of our diet.

As outlined in Part One, the Food Guide Pyramid (see chapter 2) can help children learn and a parent plan a well-balanced, healthy diet. The food pyramid has been so successful in its approach to teaching good nutrition that it has been modified to teach other areas as well. Currently, educators use variations of the Food Guide Pyramid, such as the Vegetarian Pyramid, the Mediterranean Pyramid, and even the Activity Pyramid as teaching modules. These can all help you plan your healthy lifestyles.

Healthy Eating Plan for Busy Kids

Outlined below is a suggested daily eating plan that can be modified for your busy schedule. Try to use all, or even a portion, of this guide to help you plan daily meals and snacks for the children in your home. Some parents find it helpful to create cycle menus for each day of the week, identifying Monday as pasta day, and Tuesday as chicken day, for example, in order to manage food purchasing and preparation plans. Try to find the best plan for your particular needs.

Breakfast

- cold cereal (especially whole-grain varieties) with low-fat milk
- yogurt with fresh fruit
- hot cereal (oatmeal, cream of wheat)
- waffles or pancakes with fruit topping
- whole-grain toast with fruit spread

Lunch

- sandwich of lean meat, such as turkey, roast beef, or ham, with fresh vegetables and low-fat cheese on enriched whole-grain or rye bread or roll, spread with mustard or low-fat mayonnaise

- salad (include a variety of lettuce, fresh vegetables, beans, peas, and fruits) with low-fat dressings

- soup (choose broth-based rather than cream-based)

- pasta (choose tomato-based rather than cream-based sauces)

- Hot entrée (choose baked, broiled, steamed, stewed, or roasted meat, poultry, or fish)

Dinner

- offer different hot or cold entrée selections (meat once a week, fish once or twice a week, chicken once or twice a week, pasta once or twice a week, and vegetarian once or twice a week)

- steamed vegetables and/or roasted/baked potatoes

- salad or soup (see under lunch)

Desserts

- fresh fruits
- frozen yogurt or sherbet

- low-fat cakes (angel food) with fresh fruit

Snacks

- yogurt and frozen yogurt
- fresh fruit
- low-fat cookies
- pretzels and popcorn
- vegetable sticks and dip
- graham crackers and peanut butter

What About Snacking?

There are many questions and misconceptions about snacks. Is it healthy to snack? What's the best time to snack? What's a good snack? Let's see what you think.

THE SNACKING QUIZ . . . SEE HOW YOU SNACK UP!

True or False

1. ____ For overweight children, it's best to avoid snacks and just feed them three meals a day.
2. ____ Most children do not need snacks to get the nutrition they need.
3. ____ Snacks eaten by children are typically high in fat.
4. ____ French fries are a bad snack since they are high in fat and calories.

Answers:

1. False: Three meals and two or three snacks daily are suggested for children and teens whether they are maintaining, losing, or gaining weight. Eating balanced, varied meals and snacks, in smaller portions, is the best way to obtain adequate nutrition and control weight.
2. False: Snacks may supply up to one third of a child's total calorie intake. Developing bodies need great amounts of

nutrients. Snacks help provide needed nutrition and prevent overeating at meals.

3. True: Unfortunately, the snacks most often eaten by today's kids tend to be high in fat. French fries, potato chips, chocolate, pizza, nachos, and vending machine items can do havoc to one's diet (although they can fit into a healthy diet if not chosen too frequently).

4. False: There are no good foods and bad snacks—only good and bad diets. All foods can be part of a healthy diet if eaten in *moderate* amounts. *A daily* consumption of French fries is not a healthy habit to get into, but once a week? Sure.

The best snacks are ones that are planned, and ones that offer a variety of nutrients and come from various groups of the food pyramid. But we all know children and teens are notorious for making unhealthy choices as well. A preference for soft drinks, candies, gum, cookies, and chips sometimes wins out over healthier options. These snacks come from the tip of the food pyramid, and fall into the category of empty-calorie foods, which provide little, if any, nutrition. Better snack choices would be fruits, vegetables, cheese, yogurt, and pretzels. All are from different groups within the pyramid and contribute some nutrition toward an overall daily eating plan.

FOODNOTE

Snacking is as important as the meals we eat. It's not *when* the foods are eaten that matters, it's *the foods* themselves.

Boosting Your Child's Nutrition

Preteens and teens need nutrition boosts throughout the day to help them through periods of growth spurts and high activity; few can get adequate nutrients from just three meals a day. Research has demonstrated that the body can better use the nutrients from foods eaten throughout the day than those that come from oversized meals. Snacks help by contributing to energy and nutrient needs, but in order to do so they must come from wise food choices. Up to 30 percent of a child's calories should come from snacks and should incorporate nutritious foods.

The perfect snack should be like a mini-meal: it should incorporate a small amount of carbohydrate, some protein, and a little fat as well.

Crackers with peanut butter or cheese, graham crackers with milk, and yogurt with fresh fruit are just a few examples.

WHAT'S A PARENT TO DO?

- *Offer smart snack choices* like these:
    raisins, dried fruits
    ready-to-eat cereals
    trail mixes
    peanut butter sandwiches
    low-fat cheese sticks or cubes
    graham crackers
    fresh fruits and vegetables
    yogurt or frozen yogurt
    low-fat cookies: vanilla wafers, gingersnaps, or animal crackers
    fruit-filled bars, fig bars
    baked chips
    pretzels or popcorn
    flavored rice cakes
    bagels
    breadsticks
- *Have snacks readily available* in the home for easy access.
- *Put out snacks before your child comes home from school.* A hungry child will be more likely to grab the first thing he or she sees.
- *Don't forbid any foods;* just limit them.
- *Teach moderation in snacking* as well as in meals.
- *Be a smart snacker yourself.*

Snacks are an integral part of a child's daily nutrition. It's important to offer a wide variety of healthy options and allow your children to make their own choices. As your children move through adolescence, it's inevitable that they will be drawn to the so-called empty-calorie foods that are so popular today. Forbidding these foods does *not* work, as it makes them that much *more* appealing.

As a parent, you need to teach *moderation* in terms of your snack options and encourage eating behaviors that can continue for a lifetime. This is a difficult concept to teach as well as implement for yourself.

15

SHOPPING SMART

If it is your intention to feed your family the healthiest foods you can, you may need to begin by planning what you're going to buy on your food shopping trips. No longer is it wise to stop by the grocery store on your way home from work just to pick up a few items. This usually leads to impulse buying, excess spending, and a home that never has a stock of staples.

A smart shopper is one who plans, makes lists, clips coupons, watches sale prices, shops on a full—rather than an empty—stomach, and buys nutritious, wholesome foods.

Keep your shopping as painless and stress-free as possible, too.

A SMART SHOPPER . . .

- seeks to try new recipes and makes a list of required food items
- checks food supplies on hand and keeps the freezer, refrigerator, and pantry well stocked
- keeps an ongoing list of foods needed
- uses coupons only for food items actually used
- watches store flyers for weekly specials
- shops regularly at the same store in order to learn its layout
- shops once each week in order to avoid numerous quick trips and excess spending

- shops after eating rather than before. (All foods look tempting on an empty stomach.)
- shops alone, if possible. (Although it is a good idea to occasionally involve children in food and shopping decisions, you will probably spend more when they accompany you. As a parent, use your best judgment on when it would be best to include them.)

Shopping smart minimizes stress and makes for a more pleasurable shopping experience. Once you get started, it becomes a regular part of your routine. Here are a few suggestions to help you become a smart shopper.

What to select in the store:

- lots of fruits and vegetables, especially dark green, orange, and yellow vegetables (the darker the color, the more nutritious)

- low-fat dairy foods including milk, yogurt, cheese, and cottage cheese

- lean ground beef, meats, poultry, and fish. How do you know what's lean? For meat, choose cuts like flank steak, sirloin, and tenderloin. For poultry, white meat has less fat than dark meat. For pork, choose fresh boiled ham, Canadian bacon, and pork tenderloin. Also, compare ground meat and poultry for fat content (some contain ground up skin and extra fat.) And self-basting turkeys have extra fat.

- deli-sliced lean meats, including roast beef, turkey, and ham

- frozen yogurt

- unsweetened breakfast cereals

- bagels, English muffins, rice cakes, pretzels, and biscuits. Avoid oversize muffins, bagels, and biscuits—they contain oversize portions of calories and fat.

- whole grain breads, pasta, and cereal products

- 100% whole wheat bread and grain products. (Make sure the first ingredients listed is whole wheat or *whole grain*.)

- brown rice (which offers three times the amount of fiber as white rice)

- lower-in-fat Ramen soup products (the regular versions are extra high in fat)

- canned foods without extra sugar or salt added

FOODNOTE

Be a prepared shopper. Make lists, clip coupons, and watch for store specials.

Know Your Grocery Store

It is in your best interest to take the time to learn the layout of your neighborhood grocery stores. Much research and marketing goes into placement of foods in the store. Manufacturers and storeowners will do anything possible to attract you to certain items. They bake breads and cookies to entice you, offer free samples, place packages at your (or your child's) eye level, share coupons, and add music and lights to make everything look that much better. Staple items, like milk and meats, are usually placed at the far end of the store. The reason for this is to get you to walk through the entire store in the hope that you will pick up several items on your way to the one thing you came in for. End caps, or displays at the end of the aisles, are also tempting and attractive. Sometimes these are weekly specials, but other times not. So read the signs. And the wisest tip is *learn to look up and down*. Name-brand items are placed at eye level (and these companies pay a lot of money for this placement), while store brands and generic items are placed higher and lower than eye level. It takes more effort to find these bargains. Take the time—it's worth it.

WHAT'S A PARENT TO DO?

When you have kids, whether 8 or 18 years of age, it may seem that no matter what food you buy or have at home, it's never the right thing. Here are a few ideas to help you when grocery shopping for your family.

- *Keep a pad of paper handy,* so everyone in the family can jot down what they would like you to buy when you go shopping.
- *Invite your kids to join you on shopping trips occasionally,* so they can pick out foods they like.

- *Use your freezer.* Many foods, such as sliced meats, cheeses, peanut butter, chili, breads, and sweets, freeze well. Your kids may have to use the microwave to defrost these items, but at least they will be available and you won't have to run out to buy them at an inconvenient time or when they're not on sale.
- *If you have a teenager who drives,* allow him or her to do the shopping (with a list) once in a while, to get the experience and get what he or she wants (within limits, of course).
- *Learn your supermarket's layout.*
- *Don't be tempted by attractive displays or enticing smells.* Buy only what you really want or need.
- *Watch for in-store specials.*
- *Compare prices* among name brands, store brands, and generic items.
- *Read labels for comparisons* to see if you are getting the best value.
- *Keep your home stocked with adequate staples.* This will allow you to prepare many dishes without running to the store for an item or two.
- *Resolve to consider grocery shopping a fun experience,* not a chore.
- *Go shopping when you are not in a hurry, hungry, or harried.*

Staple Items to Keep on Hand

There's nothing worse than knowing it's mealtime, you don't have any time to prepare anything, and nothing healthy is in your pantry or refrigerator. *Don't wait for this to happen.* Stocking your pantry and refrigerator is a good habit to get into. Here are some staple items to keep on hand for those occasions when time is at a minimum and hunger is not. If you can keep at least half of these items in stock, you'll have an easier time with healthy meal preparation.

For the pantry
beans, dried and canned
bouillon (chicken, vegetable, and beef)
breads, whole grain and enriched

cereal, especially bran and whole grain
crackers
dried fruits
flour, enriched and whole grain
fruits, canned in juice, without added sugar
herbs and spices
oils (corn, canola, sunflower, safflower, and/or olive)
onions
pasta, regular or whole wheat, in a variety of shapes and sizes
peanut butter
popcorn
potatoes, fresh, canned, or instant
pretzels
rice, brown and white, quick cooking
sauces (BBQ, soy, catsup, pasta)
sugar, white and brown
tomatoes, canned, whole stewed, and sauce
tuna and salmon, water-packed

For the freezer
bagels, pita bread, and other breads
boneless, skinless chicken breasts
fish fillets
frozen vegetables
frozen fruits, concentrated fruit juices
lean ground beef and other lean meats
pizza crust
frozen yogurt

For the refrigerator
canned rolls, breads, and pizza crusts
eggs
fresh fruits, in season
fresh vegetables, including lettuce, tomatoes, cucumbers, peppers,
    broccoli, and carrots
fruit juice, including citrus
low-fat milk, cheeses, yogurt, and cottage cheese
meats and poultry, lean cuts
mustard, spicy mustard
salad dressings and mayonnaise, low-fat varieties
salsa

FOODNOTE

For easy access and storage, try "pyramiding" your pantry. Store food items in your pantry in the format of the Food Guide Pyramid: grain products on the bottom shelf; canned fruits and vegetables on the next highest shelf; protein-rich foods (tuna, salmon, dried beans, dry milk powder, pudding mixes) next— and oils, fats, cookies, and candies on the less accessible top.

Remember: Keep balance, variety, and moderation when grocery shopping.

16

READING AND
UNDERSTANDING FOOD LABELS

In order for consumers to plan healthy meals and incorporate healthy foods into their diet, the Food and Drug Administration of the U.S. Department of Health and Human Services and the Food Safety and Inspection Service of the U.S. Department of Agriculture have required food manufacturers to include Nutrition Facts labels on their products since the mid-1990s. The labels tell the size or number of servings, how many calories and how much fat, cholesterol, fiber, and other nutrients are contained within each serving. Also included is information on Nutrient Reference Values (also referred to as Percentage of Daily Values). This shows what percentage of the recommended daily amount of the nutrients are provided in a serving, based on diets of 2,000 and 2,500 calories per day.

Food labels have never been easier to understand. They can help you see how healthy a particular food is, as well as how it can fit into a total diet. Here's what the label tells you:

• Serving size: These servings sizes are standardized to make it easier to compare similar products.

• Calorie and nutrition information on fat, cholesterol, sodium, total carbohydrates, and protein must be shown in grams as well as in Daily Values.

• Daily Value Percentages: This allows consumers to see how this product contributes to an overall daily diet.

This indicates the total calories and calories from fat that can be found in one serving.

These nutrients are the most important to overall health. People should try to eat 100% of the recommended daily allowance of carbohydrate, fiber, vitamins, and minerals over the period of one day. The percentages of fat, saturated fat, cholesterol and sodium should not exceed 100%.

This particular item has a serving size of 8 ounces and is 1 serving.

This information tells the % Daily Value, which is how much of the daily recommended amount of a nutrient this food supplies for a 2,000 calorie diet. One's individual daily values may vary depending on how many calories he or she needs.

Based on 2,000 calorie diets, this section indicates how much total fat, cholesterol, sodium, and carbohydrate a person needs each day.

Nutrition Facts

Serving Size 8oz. (227g)
Servings Per Container 1

Amount Per Serving

Calories 190   Calories from Fat 25

                           % Daily Value*

Total Fat 3g	**4%**
Saturated Fat 2g	**9%**
Cholesterol 10mg	**4%**
Sodium 150mg	**6%**
Total Carbohydrate 31g	**10%**
Dietary Fiber 0g	**0%**
Sugars 31g	
Protein 11g	

Vitamin A 2%	•	Vitamin C 2%
Calcium 40%	•	Iron 0%

*Percent Daily Values are based on a 2,000 calorie diet. Your daily values may be higher or lower depending on your calorie needs:

		Calories: 2,000	2,500
Total Fat	Less than	65g	80g
Saturated Fat	Less than	20g	25g
Cholesterol	Less than	300mg	300mg
Sodium	Less than	2,400mg	2,400mg
Total Carbohydrate		300g	375g
Dietary Fiber		25g	30g

Calories per gram:
     Fat 9 • Carbohydrate 4 • Protein 4

Sample Nutrition Label / Vanilla Yogurt

• Daily Values of Vitamins A and C and minerals (iron and calcium): These reveal how this food contributes to the daily diet (you and your child should aim for 100% each day).

Reading the rest of a food label can be quite confusing if you are not familiar with the lingo commonly used on food products. Here is a rundown for easy reference:

• *Calorie-free:* the product contains less than 5 calories per serving

• *Low-calorie:* the product contains 40 calories or less per serving

• *Sugar-free* or *fat-free:* the product contains less than .5 grams per serving of sugar or fat

- *Low-fat:* the product contains 3 grams or less per serving

- *Low-sodium:* the product contains 140 mg. or less per serving

- *Very low-sodium:* the product contains 35 mg. or less per serving

- *Cholesterol-free:* the product contains less than 2 mg. of cholesterol and 2 grams or less of saturated fat per serving

- *Low-cholesterol:* the product contains 20 mg. or less per serving of
cholesterol and 2 grams or less of saturated fat per serving

- *Good source:* can be used to indicate that one serving contains 10
to 19 percent of the Daily Value for a particular nutrient

- *Reduced:* can be used to indicate that one serving contains at least
25 percent less of a nutrient than the regular product

- *Lean:* can be used to indicate that a product has less than 10 grams
of fat, 4 grams of saturated fat, and 95 mg. of cholesterol per serving

- *Light:* can be used to indicate that a product has $\frac{1}{3}$ less calories and
no more than $\frac{1}{2}$ of the fat or sodium of the regular product (However,
light can sometimes refer to the *color* of the product as well.)

- *Healthy:* can be used to refer to a product that is low in fat and
saturated fat and contains limited amounts of sodium and cholesterol

---

WHAT'S A PARENT TO DO?

Keep an eye on the following details of the nutrition label for
quick information:

- *Serving size:* Pay attention to the serving size information. Is
the amount that your child would eat the same amount that
is listed?
- *Calories from fat:* Watch how many calories come from fat.
- *Dietary fiber:* Is your family reaching their daily requirement?
- *Vitamins and minerals:* Your goal here is 100 percent each day.
But don't depend on one food to do it all.
- *Remember that variety is the key.*
- *Let the Daily Value be your guide.* But remember these num-
bers are based on people who eat 2,000 and 2,500 calories

each day, *more* than what most young children consume. For fat, saturated fat, and cholesterol, choose foods with a low percentage of daily value most of the time. For total carbohydrates, dietary fiber, vitamins, and minerals, your daily value goal is to reach 100 percent of each.

FOODNOTE

Don't be overwhelmed by food labels. They were developed to help consumers choose foods more wisely and healthfully.

17

EATING OUT AND ABOUT

Eating out is a way of life today. Everyone does it in some form or another. Whether in a restaurant, a fast food drive-through, a school lunchroom, at a picnic in the park, on an airplane, in a car, or at a social or holiday event, people are eating out more today than ever before. Contributing to this increase are dual-career families, busy schedules, fatigue, and laziness. Of course, people also eat out for no other reason than just for fun. So it's no wonder that estimates indicate that at least half of all Americans eat out on a typical day.

Eating out can cause havoc to one's health, especially for people who don't have a good nutrition knowledge base. With the information provided here, you will be able to retain a good understanding of good and not-so-good choices available to you and your family when you're eating out. We're not here to tell you that eating out is bad; no, we're here to help you incorporate dining pleasures into your daily lives using some common sense and nutrition precautions.

Fast Food . . . Can It Be Healthy?

Today, fast food restaurants *are* aiming to be healthier. Many have added food choices like broiled chicken breasts, salads, baked potatoes, and tortilla wraps. It may take a little more thought on the consumer's part, however, to make the right choices. Remember that variety and moderation are the keys to eating healthily, even when it comes to fast food.

The nutrients missing from most fast food choices are vitamins A and C, the minerals iron and calcium, and fiber. By adding a salad, soup, juice, milk, low-fat yogurt shake, and/or whole grain bun or roll to your meal, these nutrients and fiber can be increased in the meal.

Put a little thought into your own or your family's fast food selections. Take a moment to think about what the rest of the day's intake was like or will be. Remember: it's the whole day's intake that counts. For example, fast foods usually contain excessive amounts of fat and salt. But if the rest of the day's intake is low in fat and sodium (salt), then a fast food meal that's higher in these nutrients is not as big of a deal. It's when no concern for the total daily intake occurs that kids and adults run the risk of developing unhealthy eating habits and health problems.

Do be cautious of the oversized portions and "combo meals" fast food restaurants offer. Even though these meals seem to be a great bargain, they are not worth the money you save when you think about how your health may be compromised.

FOODNOTE

Oversized, supersized, and "combo" meals may be cheaper, but they are not the best choice overall.

Here are a few helpful tips when it comes to ordering a fast food meal.

Instead of ordering:	Order this instead:
quarter-pounder with cheese and toppings	lean hamburger or veggie burger with pickles, mustard, catsup, and without cheese
French fries or onion rings	baked potato or salad with low-fat dressing
chicken nuggets, fish fillet, or fried or "extra crispy" chicken	broiled or grilled chicken or fish sandwich
beef burrito supreme	bean burrito or soft chicken taco

Instead of ordering:	Order this instead:
regular soda or milkshake	low-fat milk, 100% juice, low-fat frozen yogurt shake, or water
"special sauce," mayonnaise, sour cream, bacon, or extra cheese	plain, low-fat dressing, no cheese; add your own condiments
salad or salad bar with regular dressing	salad or salad bar with low-fat dressing
pie or ice cream	nonfat frozen yogurt
cream soup	low-fat soup or chili
super-sized	small size

For the leanest selections at fast food restaurants choose the following:

- Grilled chicken sandwich—plain or with low-fat toppings
- Hamburger made from lean beef or turkey, or veggie burgers (go for the small portions, as well)
- Stuffed baked potato without butter, sour cream, or cheese. Salsa is a good topping choice.
- Chicken teriyaki or fajitas, but without excess guacamole and sour cream
- Fresh meat sandwiches—roast beef, chicken, turkey, ham; hold the mayo
- Low-fat soups or chili
- Grilled or broiled chicken (skinless) in a sandwich or served with a baked potato
- Salad or salad bars with fat-free or low-fat dressing
- Water, low-fat milk, 100% fruit juice, or a low-fat shake
- Low-calorie condiments such as lower-fat mayonnaise, salad dressings, or mustard

FOODNOTE

By ordering a small vs. a supersized fries, you can save 300 to 350 calories.

The Skinny on Dining Out

Now let's see if you can figure out what's best in terms of what to order in your favorite fast food restaurant:

1. Rank the following meals from highest to lowest amount of fat:
   a. Hamburger, small fries, side salad with lite dressing, skim milk
   b. Fried chicken breast sandwich, coleslaw, mashed potatoes with gravy, cola
   c. Roast beef sandwich on wheat bun, side salad with French dressing, corn on the cob, vanilla soft serve cone, water

2. Which is the better choice at Taco Bell?
   a. taco salad
   b. big beef nachos supreme

3. Approximately how many calories can you save by eliminating the cheese from your hamburger?
   a. 50
   b. 100
   c. 150
   d. 200

4. How many calories does a personal pan cheese pizza have?
   a. 300
   b. 450
   c. 600
   d. 725

5. Which is the least caloric dessert?
   a. McDonald's ice cream cone
   b. Subway chocolate chip cookie
   c. Dairy Queen small vanilla shake
   d. Wendy's small Frosty

Answers:
1. b, a, c
2. b. The nachos have half the fat and calories as the taco salad, as of this writing.
3. b. Each piece of cheese contains about 100 calories.
4. c. You might be better off sharing the personal pan pizza or ordering 2 slices of thin and crispy cheese pizza.

5. a. As of this writing, the McDonald's ice cream cone has 150 calories (Subway cookie, 210; Dairy Queen shake, 550 calories; Wendy's Frosty, 330 calories).

FOODNOTE

Fried chicken or fish sandwiches have more fat and calories than hamburgers.

WHAT'S PARENT TO DO?

- *Set limits when it comes to choosing fast foods.* If this is impossible, go to these restaurants less frequently.
- *Have healthy sandwich supplies available at home* as an alternative to eating out at fast food restaurants.
- *Before going to the fast food restaurant,* suggest certain foods to your children that may be better choices.
- *If you take the fast food home,* add fresh fruit, vegetables, and/or milk to balance the meal.
- *Share an order of fries.*

The Secret to Restaurant Dining Success

Eating out has become a way of life, and table-service restaurants are now recognizing the concern of their patrons—particularly those who want healthier meal options. Some restaurants even mark the healthier items on the menus with a symbol or a star.

Many family restaurants are now using healthier cooking methods. In many places, menu selections are generally baked, broiled, or steamed instead of fried. More chicken, fish, salad, and vegetarian options are available and you can make substitutions for higher-fat foods. But the responsibility for healthy eating remains with the *consumer.*

Here are a few hints to making that restaurant meal a little healthier:

- Don't feel obligated to order every course. Choose soup or salad and skip dessert.

- Don't feel you have to eat everything on your plate. Portions in restaurants are larger than the average person needs—often up to four times larger! Ask for a "doggie bag." Some people ask for the doggie bag before they get their meal and put the extra food away before they begin to eat so that they don't inadvertently eat more that they wish.

- If you don't know what's in a dish, ask.

- Share your meal with another family member (if, by chance you agree on the same thing).

- Eat slowly, so your body has time to feel full (it takes twenty minutes for your stomach to signal your brain that it's full).

- Ask for your food plain, with the sauce, dressing, sour cream, or other toppings on the side. You can add them yourself, if desired, in smaller amounts than the cook would have done.

- Ask for substitutions. Instead of fried potatoes, request grilled vegetables, a plain baked potato, or fruit.

- Don't drink your calories. Ask for water with lemon, diet drinks, or unsweetened ice tea with lemon.

- Be creative. Try a lower-fat appetizer with soup or salad, instead of ordering an entrée.

- Don't order fried or breaded foods. Go for broiled, baked, or roasted options.

- Remember; *you* are the role model. You can help teach your children properly by making the right choices for yourself.

Here are some ideas on what to choose when you dine out in specialty restaurants:

Pizza Places

Beware of "deep-dish" and "grande" options, as generally these have more fat. Toppings, such as extra cheese, sausage, bacon, and pepperoni can more than double the amount of fat in each slice of pizza. Try to do without them.

Better choices would be to go light on the cheese, order no cheese, or choose low-fat mozzarella cheese, and/or a thin crust. Almost any vegetable topping, which adds some fiber and vitamins to your meal, would be fine. If a whole-wheat crust is an option, go for it! Healthier meat options would be Canadian bacon, chicken, ham, crabmeat, and shrimp. If you absolutely must have thick pizza, have less of it and take home the leftovers.

Chinese, Japanese, and Thai

Limit "crispy" or "fried" items. These fried and breaded foods are major sources of fat, which means lots of calories. Also, avoid buffets. You'll eat more than you need, and more fat is added to buffet foods so they won't stick to the pans. Sweet-and-sour items are higher in calories because of the excessive amount of sugar they contain. Nuts also add a lot of calories to foods.

Better choices include steamed rice, boiled noodles, steamed dumplings, soup (most of the soups are low in fat and calories), stir-fried vegetables or tofu, and chop suey. Ask for less oil in preparation and for more vegetables than meat in your entrée. Learn to use chopsticks—they'll slow you down.

FOODNOTE

Beware of nuts and fried noodles as toppings on Chinese foods. There are 200 calories and 20 grams of fat in $\frac{1}{4}$ cup of nuts. And 125 calories and 6 grams of fat in $\frac{1}{4}$ cup of fried noodles.

Mexican

Stay away from the many high-calorie entrées and accompaniments: chalupas, tostados, chimichangas, beef or cheese enchiladas, tamales, and tacos; sour cream, guacamole, and cheese. Also, watch how much you eat out of the basket of tortilla chips often placed in front of you on the table.

Wiser selections are the lower-calorie entrées: fajitas, soft tacos, soft burritos, chicken enchiladas, arroz con pollo (chicken with rice), and ceviche (fish). Use salsa and ask for baked tortilla chips. If you have to eat the fried chips, limit the amount you eat and then have the rest removed. Ask for beans made without lard or other fat.

Italian

Be cautious of oil and cream sauces. To eat lean, try limiting dishes with a lot of meat, cheese, and oil. Avoid fried foods, such as calamari, altogether. Eggplant, chicken, or veal parmigiana; fettuccine alfredo; and lasagna contain excessive amounts of high-fat cheese and cream sauces.

Better choices would be pasta with red or white clam sauce or marinara sauce. Choose pasta with meat rather than an entrée that's mainly meat. Choose entrées that can be steamed, grilled, or broiled instead of sautéed or fried. Avoid cheesy dishes. If you have a favorite high-fat sauce, ask for it on the side or "light on the sauce." Italian ice is a nice dessert.

Deli and Sandwich Shops

There are so many healthy options for sandwich fillings and breads these days that it's easy to choose a tasty, nutritious sandwich. To limit the amount of fat in your sandwich, order sliced roast beef, turkey, or chicken breast on whole wheat bread with tomatoes, lettuce, and other vegetables. If turkey-ham is available, this is an adequate choice, too. Request no mayonnaise, or ask for it to be on the side. The deli may carry low-fat or no-fat mayonnaise, but you have to request it. Stay away from sandwich fillings such as tuna, egg, or chicken salads—they are made with excess fat.

Remember: you don't have to eat an *entire* sandwich. Sharing may be an option, or take half home to eat later.

In a deli, you need to be aware of the side salads. If just a small amount is eaten, there's no need to worry. But many of these salads are loaded with mayonnaise—that is, fat. Also, the chips or fries that are often served with sandwiches can almost double the calorie value of the meal without adding much else. When ordering soup, go for the broth-based soups. And try vegetarian soups, such as lentil, split pea, or vegetable. It's a good way to get fiber and some often-missed vitamins and minerals.

Wherever you decide to eat out, beware of the following terms—they all mean "high in fat."

alfredo	cheesy
au gratin	scalloped
cheese sauce	pan-fried
breaded	basted
butter-dipped	crispy
fried	sautéed
creamed (or creamy)	batter-dipped
hollandaise	smothered
in gravy	stuffed
pastry	

WHAT'S A PARENT TO DO?

- *Discuss the healthier food choices with your child* before going to a particular restaurant.
- *If healthful choices are too difficult to make at a certain restaurant,* try going to one where a wider variety of options are offered.
- *If you bring home the main entrée,* add vegetables, fruit, and/or milk to balance the meal.
- *Share a meal.*
- *Ask questions as to how the food is made and if there are more nutritious options available.* Don't be afraid to make a special request. You are the paying customer.

FOODNOTE

Be sure to get what you want when eating out. You are paying for it.

Healthy Holiday Hints

Holidays are festive times to enjoy the company of friends and family, continue family traditions, and, of course, eat. But the focus should not just be on the foods. It seems when the holidays roll around, we all lose any self-control we may have had and use these times as splurge times. Still, there are simple steps you can take to make special occasions a little healthier.

Instead of:	Choose:
$\frac{1}{4}$ cup sour cream (60 calories) on potato pancakes	$\frac{1}{4}$ cup applesauce (30 calories)
meat lasagna (300 calories)	vegetable lasagna (180 calories)
turkey leg (170 calories)	turkey breast (no skin) (135 calories)
beef patty (240 calories)	veggie burger (84 calories)
pork chops (2 = 300 calories)	pork tenderloin (3 oz. = 140 calories)

Instead of:	Choose:
fried shrimp (3 = 210 calories)	6 steamed shrimp (105 calories)
candied sweet potatoes ($\frac{1}{2}$ cup = 220 calories)	baked sweet potatoes ($\frac{1}{2}$ cup = 120 calories)
stuffing inside the turkey	stuffing baked outside the turkey
supermoist cake mixes (250 calories/slice)	chiffon/angel food cake mixes (130 calories/slice)
oil, butter, or margarine in cake or bread mixes (1,000 calories/cup)	applesauce or prune puree (120 calories/cup)
sour cream in noodle kugels (60 calories)	nonfat plain yogurt (40 calories)
premium ice cream (340 calories)	low-fat frozen yogurt (200 calories)
pecan pie (450 calories/slice)	pumpkin pie (230 calories/slice)
guacamole (177 calories)	salsa (20 calories)
regular sour cream or mayonnaise (100 calories)	low-fat or fat-free sour cream or mayonnaise (50 calories)
hot buttered rum (200 calories)	hot spiced wine (100 calories)
$\frac{1}{4}$ cup hot fudge (130 calories)	2 tbsp. chocolate syrup (60 calories)

If you make some of these choices, your holidays and special occasions may be a little leaner and more nutritious.

WHAT'S A PARENT TO DO?

- *If you are celebrating the holiday meal away from home,* discuss the possibilities with your child of what may be served at the party. Make suggestions about which foods may need to be limited.
- *If you are cooking, then you'll know what's being served.* You can alter recipes to make them healthier and still taste good. You can also remind your family that there will be leftovers, so not

to worry if they can't eat as much as they want the first go-around.

- *Allow more flexible limits during holiday times.* If your family eats healthily the rest of the year, the few days of holiday celebration will not make much of a difference in their total health.
- *Do not volunteer to bring home leftover sweets or fatty leftovers.* It's too much of a temptation for most people.
- *Remember balance, moderation, and variety*—if you can.
- *Try to enjoy holiday customs* of singing, sending cards, and decorating, while putting less emphasis on eating.

Lunching at School: "To Bring or Not to Bring" Is the Question

Often, a child or teen will have a strong preference regarding buying the hot lunch at school or bringing lunch from home (although some schools may not have a hot lunch program). Lunch is only one meal, but in a student's routine, lunches at school become important influences on health and well-being.

A few words about hot lunch programs: Recently, some school systems have tried to make the hot lunch program healthier. Salad bars, fresh fruit, and low-fat and skim milk are more frequently seen. However, many schools continue to serve high-fat, high-sugar meals because that is what sells. Typical menus include chicken nuggets, pizza (sausage and pepperoni included), cheeseburgers, fried chicken, hot dogs and corn dogs, French fries, chips, fruits in heavy syrup, cookies, and cakes. Some systems have welcomed fast food chains into their schools, making cheeseburger and fries very easy to obtain. And often, limited kitchen facilities only allow schools to heat prepared, convenience-type foods rather than make meals from scratch.

If the hot lunch were the only high-fat, non-nutritious meal a child ate on a typical day, it would not be so terrible. But in today's world, where we are so busy with after school activities and parents come home from work too exhausted to cook a healthy meal, more often than not dinner becomes a fast food, convenience, or restaurant meal that is, also high in fat and low in vegetables and fruit. This is one reason we are seeing so much obesity in our kids and adults today.

It may be a wiser move to pack a lunch for your child to bring to school. Keep in mind that children from five years on up can make their own lunches (Now that's a novel idea!) When a child is involved in making a meal, which includes a packed lunch, there's a greater chance it will be eaten. Brown-bagging may save calories as well as encourage more fruits and vegetables.

Be sure to include the following in a packed lunch:

- a protein source, such as cheese, peanut butter, chicken or turkey, low-fat meats, tuna
- a fruit and/or a vegetable
- a bread or starch: whole wheat breads, crackers, bagels, or muffins are all good
- a drink: try water (or milk can be purchased at school)
- a "special something" (it could be chips occasionally, or a sweet)

Also, many kids like it when you send a thermos filled with hot foods, especially in the winter when it's colder. Soup, macaroni and cheese, and chili are a few suggestions. Here are a few more unusual but good choices to offer in the lunch box:

- meat or cheese kabobs or wraps served with fruit and milk
- cheese or meat wrapped around a pretzel, breadstick, or pickle, plus dessert and a drink
- breakfast for lunch: cereal, milk, and a banana, for example
- soup or chili in a thermos, with a bagel and fresh fruit
- leftover pizza or Chinese food
- mini drumsticks, fruit, granola bar, and milk

WHAT'S A PARENT TO DO?
- *Be sure to have enough food in the house to make healthy lunches* (see section on shopping and stocking your pantry in chapter 15).

- *Encourage variety.* Include different types of breads, fruits, desserts, as well as the main item.
- *Be flexible and allow your child to be creative.* There's no rule written in stone about what's acceptable to bring for lunch.
- *Encourage your child to prepare his or her own lunch,* but be available to help if needed.
- *Make the lunch the night before* in order to ease morning stress.
- *Make a lunchtime cycle menu* to help plan meals in advance and have appropriate supplies and foods on hand.

A word of caution on packaged lunch meals: These meals, although convenient and "cool" in appearance, are not wise choices if eaten on a regular basis. The foods included in the pack are generally high in fat, salt, food coloring, preservatives, and sugar. It would be better to buy a disposable container with separate sections and make your own lunchtime meal with fresh turkey or roast beef, crackers or pretzels, a small piece of fruit, and a miniature candy bar or two small cookies. If your child insists on these ready-made, prepackaged meals, add a fruit or a vegetable and have your child buy low-fat milk to drink. This will at least make a better-balanced meal. Also, you can limit these to one day per week as a special treat.

FOODNOTE

Remember: there is no law that says lunch must contain a sandwich. Be creative and have fun with lunch!

The Best Out-of-the-House Food Choices

Eating takes place everywhere. No longer is mealtime confined to the dining table. Food choices are made at the movies, at the mall, in school, and even in the car. All this food, whether eaten standing, sitting, or driving, adds to one's daily caloric and nutrient intake. Wise food choices need to be made everywhere. It all adds up. Here are our picks:

Where you are going	What's good to eat
The movies	fat-free candy (gummy snacks, jelly beans, licorice, sweet tarts, mints, hard

Where you are going	What's good to eat
The movies (cont.)	candy), popcorn without butter, 100% fruit juice, seltzer water, plain water, low-calorie soft drinks
Ice cream parlor	low-fat frozen yogurt, child-size cones, sorbet, sherbet, plain cones
Food court at the mall	plain soft pretzels, plain popcorn, low-fat frozen yogurt, turkey or roast beef sandwich, baked potatoes, garden salads (dressing on the side)
Vending machines	fat-free candies, pretzels, baked chips, mints, yogurt, dried fruit, trail mix, whole-grain crackers, 100% fruit juice, seltzer water, low-calorie soft drinks, water, low-fat chocolate milk
Birthday parties	baked tortilla chips with salsa, veggies and dip, crackers and cheese, fruit kabobs, plain popcorn, angel food cake, low-fat ice cream, frozen yogurt
Car trips	graham crackers, animal crackers, fresh and dried fruit, veggie sticks, pretzels, sandwiches from home

Keeping Foods Safe

Keeping foods safe falls into the hands of consumers as well as manufacturers, restaurants, and supermarkets. Safe food handling is important at all times, but particularly when foods are carried away from the refrigeration and controlled temperatures at home.

Parents should be concerned about food safety when it comes to preparing brown-bag lunches, picnics, or food for car trips. Foods carried to outdoor activities, especially during summer months, should also be packed appropriately.

Be smart when preparing and handling foods.

WHAT'S A PARENT TO DO?

- *Keep hands clean* when preparing all foods.
- *Keep hot foods hot* (use a thermos when necessary) and cold foods cold (pack appropriate ice packs, or use insulated containers).
- *Keep lunch and picnic containers out of direct sunlight,* and/or away from radiators, baseboard heaters, or other heat sources.
- *Pack mostly shelf-stable foods* (crackers, peanut butter, nonrefrigerated puddings and fruit cups).
- *Freeze juice boxes;* placed in a lunch bag, a frozen juice box will keep food cool, and be thawed in time for lunch.
- *Any perishable foods not eaten at lunch or during the outdoor activity* should be discarded.

You want your foods to be safe to eat. Never take the chance if you are not sure. "If in doubt, throw it out."

PART FOUR

RECIPES

Your family probably enjoys certain favorite and traditional foods and prepares these most often. It is easy to get into a rut and make the same foods over and over again. It is our hope that you will soon add more choices to your collection. Here we share some of our favorite kid- and family-friendly recipes to help you get started on the path toward more variety in your meals.

We have tried to address many of the common concerns discussed in this book by offering some recipes that are lower in fat and some that are higher in fat. There are higher-fiber and vegetarian recipes, favorite snacks, and more. Although any and all foods can fit into a balanced diet, recipes have been identified for your specific dietary needs. Our guidelines used are as follows:

LOWER FAT
Lower Fat = 3 grams of fat per serving or less

HIGHER FAT
Higher Fat = 8 grams of fat per serving or more

VEGETARIAN
Vegetarian Choice (Lacto-ovo Vegetarian)

HIGH-FIBER
High-Fiber Food = 2.5 grams of fiber or more

Each recipe includes a nutrient analysis listing total calories and grams of protein, carbohydrates, fat, and fiber per serving. This information can help you determine the best options for your personal needs. (Note: Optional ingredients or substitutions suggested or presented in the recipe may not be included in the overall analysis.) Analyses were completed using Food Processor Nutrition Software. Amounts listed have been rounded to the nearest value.

Recipes

DRINKS OF CHOICE

Tropical Fruit Freeze

Strawberry Banana Smoothie

Fruited Smoothie Shake

Strawberry Yogurt Smoothie

Easy Fruit Smoothie

High-Protein Breakfast Shake

Warm and Toasty Hot Chocolate

Chilled Mocha Drink

MORNING GOODNESS

Apple Cinnamon Oatmeal

Fruited Oatmeal

Fruity Breakfast Burrito

Fruity Yogurt Crunch

Spiced Apple Toast

Cinnamon Muffins

Blueberry Muffins

Applesauce Muffins

Mushroom Frittata

Challah French Toast

Overnight French Toast

Puffy German Pancake with
    Fresh Berries

Yogurt Pancakes

Warm Apple Pancake

SAVORY SOUPS AND STEWS

Very Veggie Soup

Garden Stew

Minestrone Soup

Black Bean Soup

Creamy Tomato Soup

Hearty Turkey Chili

Quick and Hearty
    Vegetarian Chili

One-Pot Vegetable Stew

SNACKING GOODIES

Zesty Bean Relish

Hummus Spread

Guacamole Olé

Munch 'N' Crunch Snack Mix

Mix & Match Trail Mix

Parmesan Tortilla Chips

Mexican Snack Mix

LUNCH AND DINNER DELIGHTS

Turkey Veggie Wrap
Wrap-a-Meal
Easy Chicken Fajitas
Southwestern Stuffed Potatoes
Black Bean Quesadillas
South of the Border Quesadillas
Barbecued Chicken Quesadillas
Pasta with Sauted Vegetables
Homemade Veggie Burgers
Turkey Burgers
Greek Pasta Stir-Fry
Spaghetti with Cherry Tomatoes
Mozzarella, Tomato,
    and Basil Couscous Salad
Pasta Alfredo
Crustless Vegetable Quiche
Baked Pasta and Cheese

Macaroni and Cheese
Spaghetti Pie
Vegetarian Pasta Bake
Broiled Pizza
Lots of Veggies Pizza
Fresh Tomato Pizza
Ratatouille
Chicken and Pasta
    with Peanut Sauce
Tuna and Cheese Pocket Melts
Cashew Chicken Casserole
Chicken Scallopini
Skillet Barbecue
Old-Fashioned Beef Stew
Easy Baked Fish Fillets

SENSATIONAL SIDES

Crispy Hash Browns
Awesome Potato Skins
Smashed Mashed Potatoes
Sweet Potato Fries
Carrot Soufflé
Pumpkin Casserole
Chinese Rice
Noodles with Peanut Sauce
Noodle Kugel

Crunchy Chicken Salad
Spinach Fruit Salad
Warm Pasta and Spinach Salad
Veggie Pasta Casserole
Broccoli and Rice Bake
Vegetable Stir-Fry with a Twist
Vegetable Chow Mein
Parmesan Couscous

BAKED BEAUTIES

Peanut Butter and Chocolate
    Chip Snackers
Banana Cake
Fruit and Cake Trifle
Peanut Butter Brownies
Apple Cake

Raspberry Yogurt Pie
Oatmeal Raisin Cookies
Low-fat Chocolate Chip Cookies
Oatmeal Chocolate Chip Cookies
Banana Chocolate Chip Bars
Apple Walnut Cookies

Lemon Glazed Zucchini Bread   Apple Crisp
Quick and Easy Zucchini Loaf .   Carrot Raisin Cake
Baked Apples

DRINKS OF CHOICE

Tropical Fruit Freeze

LOWER FAT   VEGETARIAN   HIGH-FIBER

1 frozen ripe banana (peel before freezing)
1 mango, peeled, seeded, and chopped
1 cup unsweetened pineapple juice

Combine all ingredients in a blender. Cover and blend until smooth.

Makes 2 servings
Calories: 210; Protein: 2 grams; Carbohydrates: 49 grams; Fat: 1 gram; Fiber: 3.5 grams

Strawberry Banana Smoothie

LOWER FAT   VEGETARIAN   HIGH-FIBER

1 frozen ripe banana (peel before freezing)
$\frac{1}{2}$ cup frozen strawberries
1 cup orange juice
$\frac{1}{4}$ cup plain or strawberry nonfat yogurt
1 tablespoon honey

Combine all ingredients in a blender. Cover and blend until smooth.

Makes 2 servings
Calories: 174; Protein: 3 grams; Carbohydrates: 43 grams; Fat: 1 gram; Fiber: 3 grams

Fruited Smoothie Shake

LOWER FAT   VEGETARIAN

1 8-ounce carton fruited yogurt
1 frozen ripe banana (peel before freezing) or $\frac{1}{2}$ cup frozen strawberries
$\frac{1}{2}$ cup low-fat milk
2 tablespoons wheat germ

(continued)

Combine all ingredients in a blender. Cover and blend until smooth.

Makes 2 servings
Calories: 220; Protein: 9 grams; Carbohydrates: 42 grams; Fat: 2 grams; Fiber: 2 grams

Strawberry Yogurt Smoothie

LOWER FAT   VEGETARIAN

1 frozen banana (peel before freezing)
1 cup fresh strawberries
1 8-ounce carton strawberry nonfat yogurt
1 cup low-fat milk

Combine all ingredients in a blender. Cover and blend until smooth.

Makes 4 servings
Calories: 100; Protein: 5 grams; Carbohydrates: 19 grams; Fat: 1 gram; Fiber: 2 grams

Easy Fruit Smoothie

LOWER FAT   VEGETARIAN

1 8-ounce carton vanilla yogurt
1 cup frozen fruit (banana, strawberries, raspberries, blueberries,
    peaches or any fruit of choice)

Combine all ingredients in a blender. Cover and blend until smooth.

Makes 2 servings
Calories: 150; Protein: 7 grams; Carbohydrates: 31 grams; Fat: none; Fiber: 2 grams

High-Protein Breakfast Shake

LOWER FAT   VEGETARIAN   HIGH-FIBER

1 tablespoon plain nonfat yogurt
$\frac{1}{2}$ cup orange juice
$\frac{1}{4}$ cup liquid egg substitute
$\frac{1}{2}$ cup frozen fruit (peaches or strawberries work best)

1 small frozen banana (peel before freezing)

¼ teaspoon vanilla extract

Combine all ingredients in a blender. Cover and blend until smooth.

Makes 1 serving
Calories: 262; Protein: 11 grams; Carbohydrates: 52 grams; Fat: 3 grams; Fiber: 5.5 grams

Warm and Toasty Hot Chocolate

LOWER FAT   VEGETARIAN

1 tablespoon sugar

1 tablespoon cocoa powder

1 cup skim milk or 1% milk

Place sugar and cocoa powder in a microwave-safe mug. Stir in a little milk to make a paste. Add remaining milk. Microwave for 1½ minutes. Stir before drinking.

Makes 1 serving
Calories: 146; Protein: 9 grams; Carbohydrates: 27 grams; Fat: 1 gram; Fiber: none

Chilled Mocha Drink

VEGETARIAN

1 cup low-fat milk

⅓ cup brewed coffee

1 teaspoon sugar

1 ounce chopped bittersweet chocolate

Combine all ingredients in a blender. Blend until well mixed. Pour into glasses filled with ice.

Makes 2 servings
Calories: 143; Protein: 6 grams; Carbohydrates: 17 grams; Fat: 6 grams; Fiber: 1 gram

MORNING GOODNESS

Apple Cinnamon Oatmeal

LOWER FAT   VEGETARIAN   HIGH-FIBER

1 cup cooked oatmeal
$\frac{1}{4}$ cup applesauce
$\frac{1}{2}$ teaspoon cinnamon
$\frac{1}{4}$ teaspoon nutmeg

Combine all ingredients in small bowl. Mix well. Divide into cereal bowls to serve.

Makes 2 servings
Calories: 89; Protein: 3 grams; Carbohydrates: 17 grams; Fat: 1 gram; Fiber: 2.5 grams

Fruited Oatmeal

LOWER FAT   VEGETARIAN   HIGH-FIBER

3 cups low-fat milk or water
1 cup rolled oats
1 apple, peeled and chopped
$\frac{1}{2}$ cup raisins
1 teaspoon cinnamon

In large saucepan, heat milk over medium heat until it begins to boil. Add remaining ingredients. Reduce heat and cook, approximately 5 minutes, until oatmeal thickens. Stir frequently to prevent sticking. Serve warm.

Makes 4 servings
Calories: 234; Protein: 10 grams; Carbohydrates: 43 grams; Fat: 3 grams; Fiber: 5 grams

Fruity Breakfast Burrito

LOWER FAT   VEGETARIAN   HIGH-FIBER

1 8-inch flour tortilla
1 teaspoon strawberry fruit spread
1 teaspoon sugar
$\frac{1}{4}$ teaspoon cinnamon
dash nutmeg
1 small banana

Place tortilla on plate. Cover with fruit spread. Sprinkle with sugar, cinnamon, and nutmeg. Place banana in center of tortilla and roll up.

Makes 1 burrito
Calories: 232; Protein: 6 grams; Carbohydrates: 48 grams; Fat: 3 grams; Fiber: 3 grams

Fruity Yogurt Crunch

LOWER FAT   VEGETARIAN   HIGH-FIBER

$\frac{1}{2}$ cup low-fat granola

1 8-ounce carton low-fat vanilla yogurt

$\frac{1}{2}$ cup crushed pineapple

$\frac{1}{2}$ cup chopped mango slices

Sprinkle half of the granola into the bottom of 2 small bowls, reserving the remaining half for topping. Evenly divide yogurt and fruit between the 2 bowls. Top with reserved granola.

Makes 2 servings
Calories: 247; Protein: 7 grams; Carbohydrates: 51 grams; Fat: 3 grams; Fiber: 2.5 grams

Spiced Apple Toast

LOWER FAT   VEGETARIAN   HIGH-FIBER

6 pieces whole wheat toast

2 apples, thinly sliced

1 tablespoon margarine

1 tablespoon brown sugar

$\frac{1}{2}$ teaspoon cinnamon

Place a few apple slices on each piece of toast and dot with margarine. Sprinkle with brown sugar and cinnamon. Place under broiler until margarine melts.

Makes 6 servings
Calories: 114; Protein: 2 grams; Carbohydrates: 21 grams; Fat: 3 grams; Fiber: 3 grams

Cinnamon Muffins

HIGHER FAT   VEGETARIAN

vegetable oil cooking spray

$1\frac{3}{4}$ cup all-purpose flour

$1\frac{1}{2}$ teaspoons baking powder

$\frac{1}{2}$ teaspoon salt

$\frac{1}{2}$ teaspoon cinnamon

$\frac{1}{4}$ teaspoon nutmeg

$\frac{1}{3}$ cup vegetable oil

$\frac{3}{4}$ cup sugar

1 egg

$\frac{3}{4}$ cup low-fat milk

Topping:

$\frac{1}{2}$ cup sugar

2 teaspoons cinnamon

2 tablespoons melted margarine

Preheat oven to 350°F. Spray muffin tin with cooking spray.

Combine flour, baking powder, salt, cinnamon, and nutmeg in medium bowl. In large bowl, combine oil and sugar. Add egg and mix well. Stir in dry ingredients alternately with milk.

Pour batter into muffin cups. Bake 20 to 25 minutes or until golden brown and a toothpick inserted into muffin comes out clean.

Combine sugar and cinnamon for topping. Brush warm muffins with melted margarine.

Sprinkle with sugar-cinnamon mixture.

Makes 1 dozen muffins
(Per Muffin) Calories: 236; Protein: 3 grams; Carbohydrates: 36 grams; Fat: 9 grams;
Fiber: none

Blueberry Muffins

VEGETARIAN

vegetable oil cooking spray

$1\frac{1}{4}$ cup plus 1 teaspoon sugar

$\frac{1}{3}$ cup vegetable oil

2 eggs

2 cups all-purpose flour

2 teaspoons baking powder

½ teaspoon salt

½ cup low-fat milk

2 cups fresh blueberries

Preheat oven to 375°F. Spray muffin tin with cooking spray.

With an electric mixer on low speed, blend 1¼ cups sugar and oil until fluffy. Add eggs, one at a time, and mix thoroughly. In a separate bowl, sift together the flour, baking powder, and salt. Add to sugar/oil mixture alternately with milk.

Mash half of the blueberries and stir in by hand. Add the remaining whole blueberries and stir in by hand.

Pour batter into muffin cups, almost to the top. Sprinkle with 1 teaspoon sugar. Bake 25 to 30 minutes or until light golden brown and a toothpick inserted into muffin comes out clean.

Makes 1 dozen muffins
(Per muffin) Calories: 236; Protein: 3 grams; Carbohydrates: 40 grams; Fat: 7 grams;
Fiber: 1 gram

Applesauce Muffins

VEGETARIAN

vegetable oil cooking spray

1½ cups all purpose flour

1 teaspoon baking powder

½ teaspoon baking soda

1 teaspoon cinnamon

½ teaspoon nutmeg

½ teaspoon salt

4 tablespoons margarine, melted

2 eggs

½ cup brown sugar

1½ cups chunky applesauce

Preheat oven to 375°F. Spray muffin tin with cooking spray.

Combine flour, baking powder, baking soda, cinnamon, nutmeg, and salt in large mixing bowl.

(continued)

In another large bowl, combine melted margarine, eggs, brown sugar, and applesauce. Mix well.

Pour the applesauce mixture into the flour mixture and stir with a wooden spoon until flour is completely absorbed.

Pour batter into each muffin cup, almost to the top. Bake 20 minutes or until light brown and toothpick inserted into muffin comes out clean.

Makes 1 dozen
(Per muffin) Calories: 155; Protein: 3 grams; Carbohydrates: 25 grams; Fat: 5 grams; Fiber: .5 gram

Mushroom Frittata

HIGHER FAT   VEGETARIAN

4 eggs, beaten (or 1 cup egg substitute to reduce total fat)

$\frac{1}{4}$ cup part-skim mozzarella or low-fat cheddar cheese

$\frac{1}{4}$ cup sliced mushrooms

1 tablespoon margarine

Preheat broiler.

In medium bowl, combine eggs, cheese, and mushrooms.

Melt margarine in oven-proof skillet over medium heat. Pour egg mixture into skillet and cook until bottom is formed and golden brown, about 5 to 6 minutes.

Remove skillet from heat and place under broiler for 1 to 2 minutes or until top becomes puffy and light brown. Remove from broiler, cool slightly, and cut into wedges to serve.

Makes 2 servings
Calories: 238; Protein: 16 grams; Carbohydrates: 2 grams; Fat: 18 grams; Fiber: none

Challah French Toast

HIGHER FAT   VEGETARIAN

4 eggs, beaten (or 1 cup egg substitute to reduce total fat)

1 cup low-fat milk

$\frac{1}{2}$ teaspoon vanilla extract

$\frac{1}{2}$ teaspoon cinnamon

$\frac{1}{4}$ teaspoon nutmeg

3 tablespoons margarine

12 slices day-old or stale Challah or other egg bread

¼ cup confectioners' sugar, optional

fresh berries, optional

In medium bowl, combine eggs, milk, vanilla, cinnamon, and nutmeg.

Heat margarine in skillet over medium heat.

Dip bread slices in egg mixture and place in heated skillet. Cook bread about 1 to 2 minutes on each side until light brown.

Sprinkle with confectioners' sugar or fresh berries, if desired.

Makes 6 servings

Calories: 331; Protein: 13 grams; Carbohydrates: 41 grams; Fat: 12 grams; Fiber: 2 grams

Overnight Baked French Toast

VEGETARIAN   HIGH-FIBER

vegetable oil cooking spray

1 small loaf whole wheat bread, cut into 1-inch cubes (or use any
　　bread of your choice)

4 eggs (or 1 cup egg substitute to reduce total fat)

3 cups low-fat milk

1 teaspoon vanilla extract

½ teaspoon cinnamon

¼ teaspoon nutmeg

Topping:

2 tablespoons margarine

2 tablespoons maple syrup

½ cup brown sugar

Spray a 9-by-13-inch baking pan with cooking spray. Spread bread cubes in a single layer in pan. In large bowl, whisk together eggs, milk, vanilla, cinnamon, and nutmeg. Pour mixture over bread cubes, making sure all the bread is well-soaked. Cover tightly and refrigerate overnight.

In the morning, preheat oven to 350°F. Melt margarine in small saucepan. Add syrup and brown sugar and mix thoroughly. Pour syrup mixture over bread. Bake for 30 to 35 minutes. Serve warm.

Makes 10 servings

Calories: 246; Protein: 10 grams; Carbohydrates: 38 grams; Fat: 7 grams; Fiber: 3 grams

Puffy German Pancake with Fresh Berries

VEGETARIAN

1 tablespoon margarine

3 eggs, beaten

⅔ cup low-fat milk

¾ cup all-purpose flour

½ teaspoon vanilla extract

½ teaspoon salt

1 cup fresh berries, raspberries, blueberries, strawberries

1 tablespoon confectioners' sugar

Preheat oven to 450°F.

Melt margarine in a 9-inch glass pie pan in oven.

In large bowl, combine eggs, milk, flour, vanilla, and salt. Whisk until well combined.

Pour batter into pie pan. Bake 12 minutes or until puffy and light brown. Remove from oven. Cool slightly.

Fill center of pancake with fresh berries and sprinkle with confectioner's sugar before serving.

Makes 4 servings

Calories: 214; Protein: 9 grams; Carbohydrates: 27 grams; Fat: 7 grams; Fiber: 2 grams

Yogurt Pancakes

VEGETARIAN

1 egg

¾ cup plain nonfat yogurt

¾ cup low-fat milk

¾ cup flour

1 teaspoon vanilla extract

1 tablespoon vegetable oil

syrup (optional)

Combine egg with yogurt and mix well. Stir in milk, flour, and vanilla. Mix until batter is smooth. Heat oil in skillet. Drop heaping spoonfuls of batter into skillet. Cook 1 minute on each side until golden brown. Serve with syrup, if desired.

Makes 4 servings

Calories: 177; Protein: 8 grams; Carbohydrates: 25 grams; Fat: 5 grams; Fiber: none

Warm Apple Pancake

VEGETARIAN

4 tart apples, peeled, cored, and thinly sliced

$\frac{1}{4}$ cup brown sugar

$\frac{1}{4}$ cup lemon juice

vegetable oil cooking spray

1 cup all-purpose flour

1 cup low-fat milk

3 tablespoons sugar

3 eggs

2 teaspoons margarine

1 tablespoon confectioners' sugar, optional

Preheat oven to 425°F.

Combine sliced apples, brown sugar, and lemon juice in a small bowl. Spray oven-proof skillet with cooking spray and heat over medium heat. Add apple mixture and sauté 3 to 5 minutes or until apples are golden brown. Remove apple mixture and set aside (do not clean skillet).

Put flour into a large bowl. In another bowl, combine milk, sugar, and eggs and mix thoroughly. Add milk mixture to flour and stir until well blended.

Melt margarine in the oven-proof skillet. Pour batter into skillet. Bake 25 minutes or until pancake is puffy and golden brown. Remove from oven. Top with apple mixture. Return to oven for 1 or 2 minutes to warm. Remove from oven and top with confectioners' sugar, if desired. Serve immediately.

Makes 6 servings

Calories: 257; Protein: 7 grams; Carbohydrates: 48 grams; Fat: 5 grams; Fiber: 2 grams

SAVORY SOUPS AND STEWS

Very Veggie Soup

LOWER FAT   VEGETARIAN   HIGH-FIBER

4 cups water

3 vegetable, chicken, or beef bouillon cubes

2 carrots, cut into 1-inch pieces

(continued)

1 onion, chopped

1 medium potato, chopped

1 15-ounce can stewed tomatoes, chopped

1 teaspoon pepper

2 cloves garlic, minced

1 bay leaf

Optional: up to 1 cup total of chopped broccoli, cabbage, corn, cauliflower, zucchini and/or beans; $\frac{1}{4}$ cup uncooked pasta and/or rice
(Note: If adding pasta or rice, increase water to $4\frac{1}{2}$ cups)

Combine all ingredients in a 4-quart pot and bring to a boil.
Reduce heat and simmer for 1 hour or until vegetables are tender.

Makes 4 servings
Calories: 110; Protein: 3 grams; Carbohydrates: 24 grams; Fat: none; Fiber: 3 grams

Garden Stew

LOWER FAT   VEGETARIAN   HIGH-FIBER

10 mushrooms fresh or canned, sliced

1 large onion, chopped

1 clove garlic, minced

5 medium zucchini, halved lengthwise and sliced

1 large eggplant, cut into 1-inch cubes

1 15-ounce can tomatoes, peeled and without seasonings

2 6-ounce cans tomato paste

$\frac{1}{2}$ medium green bell pepper, seeded and diced

1 teaspoon salt

1 teaspoon thyme

1 teaspoon basil

1 teaspoon oregano

$\frac{1}{4}$ teaspoon pepper

In large soup pot or Dutch oven, combine all ingredients. Cook
uncovered on low heat until the vegetables soften and liquid thickens,
about $1\frac{1}{2}$ to 2 hours.

Makes 6 servings
Calories: 115; Protein: 6 grams; Carbohydrates: 26 grams; Fat: 1 gram; Fiber: 7 grams

Minestrone Soup

LOWER FAT   VEGETARIAN   HIGH-FIBER

9 cups water

2 teaspoons vegetable oil

2 cloves garlic, peeled and minced

1 small onion, chopped

1 6-ounce can tomato paste

2 teaspoons dried basil

$\frac{1}{2}$ teaspoon pepper

1 16-ounce can kidney beans, drained and washed

4 cups mixed chopped vegetables, (zucchini, green beans, carrots, cabbage)

1 potato, peeled and diced, optional

1 cup uncooked macaroni

Heat water in large saucepan or Dutch oven. Heat oil in a small skillet, and sauté garlic and onion. Add to water. Add tomato paste, basil, pepper, kidney beans, and all of the vegetables, including potatoes, if using. Bring to boil. Add macaroni. Reduce heat and simmer, uncovered for 20 to 30 minutes until pasta is cooked and vegetables are tender. Remove from heat. Cool slightly before serving.

Makes 10 servings

Calories: 146; Protein: 6 grams; Carbohydrates: 28 grams; Fat: 1 gram; Fiber: 6 grams

Black Bean Soup

LOWER FAT   VEGETARIAN   HIGH-FIBER

3 15-ounce cans black beans, drained and rinsed, separated

1 teaspoon vegetable oil

1 medium onion, chopped

2 cloves garlic, minced

1 green pepper, seeded and chopped

3 cups vegetable broth

$1\frac{1}{2}$ cups chopped fresh tomatoes (about 3 tomatoes)

1 teaspoon cumin

1 teaspoon oregano

(continued)

In food processor, puree 2 cans of the black beans with $\frac{1}{2}$ cup water.

Heat oil in large saucepan. Add onion, garlic, and green pepper. Cook until tender. Add bean puree, remaining can of beans with 2 cups water, vegetable broth, tomatoes, cumin, and oregano. Bring to a boil, then reduce heat, cover, and simmer 20 minutes.

Makes 6 servings
Calories: 207; Protein: 13 grams; Carbohydrates: 35 grams; Fat: 3 grams; Fiber: 13 grams

Creamy Tomato Soup

LOWER FAT   VEGETARIAN

2 tomatoes, peeled and chopped
$1\frac{1}{2}$ cups tomato juice
1 tablespoon dried basil
$\frac{1}{2}$ cup low-fat milk
$\frac{1}{4}$ teaspoon salt
$\frac{1}{4}$ teaspoon pepper
2 ounces softened low-fat cream cheese

In medium saucepan, combine tomatoes and tomato juice. Bring to a boil, then reduce heat and simmer 30 minutes, uncovered.

Place tomato mixture in food processor or blender. Process until smooth. Return mixture to saucepan. Add basil, milk, salt, pepper, and cream cheese. Over medium heat, stir well with a whisk until all ingredients are well mixed and soup begins to thicken.

Makes 4 servings
Calories: 71; Protein: 4 grams; Carbohydrates: 7 grams; Fat: 3 grams; Fiber: 1 gram

Hearty Turkey Chili

HIGH-FIBER

vegetable oil cooking spray
1 pound lean ground turkey
1 15-ounce can kidney beans
1 16-ounce can stewed tomatoes
1 6-ounce can tomato paste
2 tablespoons chili powder
2 tablespoons minced onion
$\frac{1}{2}$ teaspoon garlic powder

$\frac{1}{2}$ teaspoon oregano

$\frac{1}{2}$ teaspoon cumin

$\frac{1}{2}$ teaspoon paprika

$\frac{1}{2}$ teaspoon salt

dash black pepper

Spray large saucepan or Dutch oven with cooking spray. Crumble ground turkey into saucepan and cook 3 to 4 minutes or until browned. Add 2 cups water and remaining ingredients. Bring to a boil, then reduce heat and simmer, uncovered, for 20 minutes or until water has evaporated and chili has thickened.

Makes 6 servings

Calories: 218; Protein: 19 grams; Carbohydrates: 22 grams; Fat: 7 grams; Fiber: 5 grams

Quick and Hearty Vegetarian Chili

LOWER FAT   VEGETARIAN   HIGH-FIBER

1 tablespoon vegetable oil

1 large onion, chopped

3 cloves garlic, minced

1 large green bell pepper, seeded and chopped

1 large red bell pepper, seeded and chopped

1 medium zucchini, diced

1 medium yellow squash, diced

1 14-ounce can diced seasoned tomatoes, undrained

1 8$\frac{3}{4}$-ounce can corn, drained

1 15-ounce can kidney beans, undrained

1 15-ounce can black beans, undrained

1 15-ounce can pinto beans, undrained

1 tablespoon chili powder

Heat oil in large skillet over medium heat. Add onion and garlic and sauté for 1 minute until tender. Add remaining vegetables and beans. Sauté several minutes more. Stir in chili powder. Reduce heat to low. Simmer, uncovered, for 20 to 30 minutes until vegetables and beans are tender and chili is thickened.

Makes 8 servings

Calories: 230; Protein: 12 grams; Carbohydrates: 40 grams; Fat: 3 grams; Fiber: 13 grams

One-Pot Vegetable Stew

LOWER FAT   VEGETARIAN   HIGH-FIBER

1 zucchini, shredded

1 carrot, shredded

1 onion, finely chopped

1 green bell pepper, seeded and chopped

1 16-ounce can stewed tomatoes, chopped

1 4-ounce can tomato sauce

1 cup hot water

1 15-ounce can kidney beans

1 packet chili seasoning

1 6-ounce package frozen hash brown potatoes

1 cup shredded low-fat cheddar cheese, optional

Combine all ingredients except cheese in large saucepan or Dutch oven. Bring to a boil, then reduce heat and simmer 20 to 30 minutes until vegetables and potatoes are tender, stirring occasionally. Before serving, top with cheese, if desired.

Makes 6 servings
Calories: 186; Protein: 12 grams; Carbohydrates: 32 grams; Fat: 2 grams; Fiber: 10 grams

SNACKING GOODIES

Zesty Bean Relish

LOWER FAT   VEGETARIAN

2 15-ounce cans black-eyed peas, drained and rinsed

1 cup chopped green onion

1 cup chopped white onion

1 cup chopped bell pepper (use combination of red, green and yellow, if desired)

$\frac{1}{4}$ cup chopped jalapeno pepper

1 2-ounce jar pimentos

1 16-ounce bottle light Zesty Italian Dressing

garlic powder, salt, pepper to taste

Combine all ingredients in large bowl. Chill until ready to serve. Serve with crackers or with chicken and fish dishes.

Makes 24 ($\frac{1}{4}$ -cup) servings
Calories: 55; Protein: 2 grams; Carbohydrates: 7 grams; Fat: 2 grams; Fiber: 2 grams

Hummus Spread

VEGETARIAN

1 15-ounce can chickpeas, drained

2 garlic cloves, crushed

$\frac{1}{4}$ cup lemon juice

$\frac{1}{4}$ cup tahini paste

$1\frac{1}{2}$ tablespoons olive oil

Place all ingredients, except olive oil, in blender. Blend until creamy, then transfer to a bowl. Pour olive oil over top to keep the hummus spread smooth and moist.

Serve with pita bread wedges or crackers.

Makes 12 (2-tablespoon) servings
Calories: 89; Protein: 3 grams; Carbohydrates: 9 grams; Fat: 5 grams; Fiber: 2 grams

Guacamole Olé

HIGHER FAT   VEGETARIAN   HIGH-FIBER

4 ripe avocados

2 tablespoons fresh lemon juice

1 tomato, peeled and finely chopped

1 whole green chili, chopped (use more if desired)

2 green onions, chopped

salt, pepper, garlic powder to taste, optional

Peel, seed, and mash avocados. In large bowl, combine avocados with lemon juice, tomato, green chili, onions, and seasonings. Mix all ingredients together with a large spoon to keep chunky or in a blender to make smoother. (To prevent browning, place avocado seed on top of mixture and cover with plastic wrap until ready to serve. Do not make guacamole more than 4 hours before serving.)

Makes about 16 ($\frac{1}{4}$ -cup) servings
Calories: 83; Protein: 1 gram; Carbohydrates: 4 grams; Fat: 8 grams; Fiber: 3 grams

Munch 'N' Crunch Snack Mix

VEGETARIAN   HIGH-FIBER

3 cups unsweetened ready-to-eat cereal

1 cup pretzels (any shape)

$\frac{1}{2}$ cup peanuts (or other nuts, if you prefer)

2 tablespoons vegetable oil

1 tablespoon Worcestershire sauce

1 cup raisins

1 cup dried apricots or dried apples

$\frac{1}{2}$ cup chocolate chips, optional

Preheat oven to 350°F.

Spread cereal, pretzels, and nuts in a 9-by-13-inch baking pan. In small bowl, mix together oil and Worcestershire sauce. Sprinkle over cereal mixture. Bake 10 minutes. Cool. Add fruit and chocolate chips, if desired.

Makes about 14 ($\frac{1}{2}$-cup) servings
Calories: 143; Protein: 3 grams; Carbohydrates: 23 grams; Fat: 5 grams; Fiber: 2.5 grams

Mix & Match Trail Mix

VEGETARIAN

Start with:	Add:	Add more:
toasted oat cereal	raisins	chocolate chips
fish crackers	dried cranberries	fruit snacks
mini graham crackers	dried cherries	peanuts
cheese crackers	pretzels	sunflower seeds
oyster crackers	popcorn	mini M & M candies

(The nutritional analysis is based on 1 cup toasted oat cereal, 1 cup fish crackers, $\frac{1}{2}$ cup raisins, and $\frac{1}{2}$ cup chocolate chips.)

Makes 6 ($\frac{1}{2}$-cup) servings
Calories: 177; Protein: 3 grams; Carbohydrates: 29 grams; Fat: 6 grams; Fiber: 1.5 grams

Parmesan Tortilla Chips

VEGETARIAN

4 8-inch soft tortillas

1 tablespoon vegetable oil

2 teaspoons grated Parmesan cheese

Preheat broiler.

Using a pizza cutter, kitchen scissors, or sharp knife, cut each tortilla into 8 wedges. Lightly brush both sides of all wedges with oil. Place on cookie sheet. Broil for 1 or 2 minutes on each side until lightly browned. Remove from oven. Sprinkle with Parmesan cheese while warm.

Makes 4 servings
Calories: 181; Protein: 5 grams; Carbohydrates: 25 grams; Fat: 7 grams; Fiber: none

Mexican Snack Mix

VEGETARIAN

1 tablespoon margarine

1 teaspoon chili powder

$\frac{1}{2}$ teaspoon cumin

dash garlic powder

1 cup cheese snack crackers

1 cup pretzels

1 cup oyster crackers

$\frac{1}{3}$ cup lightly salted dry-roasted nuts

$\frac{1}{2}$ cup seedless raisins

Preheat oven to 300°F.

Melt margarine in 9-by-13-inch baking pan. Remove from oven. Stir in chili powder, cumin, and garlic powder. Add crackers, pretzels, and nuts. Toss until well coated. Bake 15 minutes, stirring every 5 minutes. Remove from oven. Stir in raisins. Spread out onto paper towel to cool.

Makes about 8 ($\frac{1}{2}$-cup) servings
Calories: 167; Protein: 4 grams; Carbohydrates: 23 grams; Fat: 7 grams; Fiber: 2 grams

LUNCH AND DINNER DELIGHTS

Turkey Veggie Wrap

HIGHER FAT   HIGH-FIBER

2 10-inch tortillas
1 tablespoon low-fat mayonnaise
$\frac{1}{4}$ cup shredded lettuce
$\frac{1}{2}$ tomato, very thinly sliced
$\frac{1}{4}$ cucumber, very thinly sliced
$\frac{1}{4}$ pound thinly sliced deli turkey

Place tortillas flat on plate. Spread mayonnaise over each tortilla. Divide lettuce, tomato, and cucumber evenly and lay across tortillas. Add sliced turkey. Roll up tortillas. Seal seam with additional mayonnaise or with toothpick.

Makes 2 servings
Calories: 313; Protein: 16 grams; Carbohydrates: 44 grams; Fat: 8 grams; Fiber: 3 grams

Wrap-a-Meal

LOWER FAT   VEGETARIAN   HIGH-FIBER

Type of Wrapper	Filling	Vegetables	Topping
tortilla:	chopped	shredded lettuce	salsa
whole wheat	cooked chicken	chopped tomatoes	mayonnaise
white	chopped cooked	shredded carrots	sour cream
corn	beef	shredded zucchini	guacamole
spinach	vegetarian	onions/green onions	hot sauce
sun-dried	"ground beef"	corn	
tomato	turkey slices	mushrooms	
lettuce leaf	beans, refried,	chopped broccoli	
cabbage leaf	black, pinto	chopped avocado	
flattened	cheese, shredded or		
bread slice	grated, any variety		

Lay out a choice of wrapper. Top with your choice of filling, vegetables, and topping, and roll up. Heat, if desired.

(The nutritional analysis is based on 1 whole wheat tortilla; $\frac{1}{4}$ cup chopped boneless, skinless chicken; $\frac{1}{2}$ cup shredded lettuce; $\frac{1}{4}$ cup chopped tomatoes; 1 tablespoon salsa.)

Makes 1 serving
Calories: 156; Protein: 14 grams; Carbohydrates: 24 grams; Fat: 3 grams; Fiber: 3 grams

Easy Chicken Fajitas

HIGHER FAT   HIGH-FIBER

2 boneless, skinless chicken breasts
$\frac{1}{2}$ cup prepared salsa
$\frac{1}{2}$ cup nonfat sour cream
6 10-inch flour tortillas
1 tablespoon vegetable oil
$\frac{1}{4}$ cup chopped green bell pepper
$\frac{1}{4}$ cup chopped red bell pepper
$\frac{1}{4}$ cup chopped onion
$\frac{1}{4}$ cup chopped tomato
$\frac{1}{2}$ cup chopped lettuce
$\frac{3}{4}$ cup low-fat shredded Cheddar cheese

Bake, broil, or boil chicken breasts until cooked thoroughly. (If baking, cook at 350°F for 40 minutes.) Chop into cubes.

In small bowl, combine salsa and sour cream. Spread over each tortilla. Heat oil in medium skillet. Sauté peppers, onion, and tomato until vegetables are tender. Divide equally over tortillas. Top with lettuce, cheese, and chicken. Roll up and serve.

Makes 6 servings
Calories: 295; Protein: 25 grams; Carbohydrates: 26 grams; Fat: 9 grams; Fiber: 1 gram

Southwestern Stuffed Potatoes

HIGHER FAT   VEGETARIAN   HIGH-FIBER

2 medium baking potatoes
1 tablespoon vegetable oil
1 onion, chopped
2 tablespoons vegetarian refried beans
1 teaspoon taco seasoning
1 tomato, chopped

(continued)

2 tablespoons shredded Cheddar cheese

2 tablespoons sour cream, optional

Preheat oven to 400°F.

Bake potatoes for 1 hour until soft. Let cool 20 to 30 minutes.

Heat oil in medium skillet. Add onions and stir-fry until tender. Add beans and taco seasoning. Cook until well heated.

Slice each potato lengthwise. Top with onion-bean mixture. Add chopped tomatoes and shredded cheese. Return to oven for 5 minutes until heated through and cheese is melted. Serve with sour cream on the side if desired.

Makes 2 servings
Calories: 272; Protein: 7 grams; Carbohydrates: 45 grams; Fat: 8 grams; Fiber: 5 grams

Black Bean Quesadillas

LOWER FAT   VEGETARIAN   HIGH-FIBER

2 10-inch flour tortillas

½ cup canned black beans

1 tablespoon salsa

1 tablespoon green onions, chopped

1 tablespoon low-fat sour cream

2 tablespoons low-fat shredded cheese, any flavor

vegetable oil cooking spray

Preheat oven to 325°F.

Spread black beans on 1 tortilla. Add remaining ingredients. Place second tortilla on top and press down.

Place on cookie sheet sprayed with cooking spray. Cook for 5 to 7 minutes, turn over, and cook an additional 5 to 7 minutes until both sides are browned and cheese is melted. Transfer to plate and cut into 4 wedges.

Makes 4 quesadilla wedges
Calories: 154; Protein: 6 grams; Carbohydrates: 25 grams; Fat: 3 grams; Fiber: 3 grams

South of the Border Quesadillas

LOWER FAT   VEGETARIAN

8 10-inch flour tortillas (try whole wheat tortillas for extra fiber)
1 15-ounce can vegetarian refried beans
1 cup shredded cheese (part-skim mozzarella, Monterey jack,
   or Cheddar)
vegetable oil cooking spray
$\frac{3}{4}$ cup salsa
optional add-ins: olives, tomatoes, sour cream, guacamole

Preheat oven to 325°F.

Spread 2 to 3 tablespoons refried beans on each of 4 tortillas and sprinkle with $\frac{1}{4}$ cup cheese. If optional ingredients are used, add them here. Place another tortilla on top and press down. Place on cookie sheet sprayed with cooking spray. Bake for 5 to 7 minutes, turn over, and bake an additional 5 to 7 minutes until both sides are browned and cheese is melted. Transfer to plate and cut into 4 wedges. Serve with salsa as a dip.

Makes 16 quesadilla wedges (1 wedge per serving for children;
2 wedges per serving for teens)
Calories: 117; Protein: 5 grams; Carbohydrates: 17 grams; Fat: 3 grams; Fiber: 1.5 grams

Barbecued Chicken Quesadillas

1 tablespoon vegetable oil
2 skinless, boneless chicken breasts, cut into strips
$\frac{1}{4}$ cup bottled barbecue sauce
$\frac{1}{2}$ cup chopped tomato
$\frac{1}{4}$ cup chopped onion
4 10-inch flour tortillas (try whole wheat tortillas for extra fiber)
$\frac{1}{4}$ cup shredded cheese, any type
vegetable oil cooking spray

Preheat oven to 325°F.

Heat oil in medium skillet. Add chicken and sauté, stirring occasionally, about 5 to 6 minutes. Remove from heat. Toss with barbecue sauce.

(continued)

Combine tomato and onion in small bowl. Spoon half of the chicken mixture on to two tortillas. Top with tomato mixture and sprinkle with cheese. Top each tortilla with another tortilla and press down. Place on cookie sheet sprayed with cooking spray. Bake 5 to 7 minutes or until browned and cheese is melted. Transfer to plate and cut each into 4 wedges.

Makes 8 quesadilla wedges (1 wedge per serving for children,
2 wedges per serving for teens)
Calories: 172; Protein: 17 grams; Carbohydrates: 15 grams; Fat: 5 grams; Fiber: none

Pasta with Sautéed Vegetables

VEGETARIAN   HIGH-FIBER

8 ounces uncooked pasta, any type

1 tablespoon vegetable oil

1 eggplant, cut into $\frac{1}{4}$-inch slices

2 zucchini, cut into $\frac{1}{4}$-inch slices

1 red bell pepper, thinly sliced

2 spring onions, chopped

$\frac{1}{4}$ cup black olives, sliced

2 plum tomatoes, thinly sliced

$\frac{1}{2}$ teaspoon fresh basil, chopped

$\frac{1}{4}$ cup grated Parmesan cheese

Cook pasta according to package directions. While pasta is cooking, heat oil in large skillet. Sauté eggplant, zucchini, pepper, onion, and olives until tender. Add tomato slices and basil.

Drain pasta and toss with vegetables. Sprinkle Parmesan cheese on top. Serve immediately.

Makes 4 servings
Calories: 223; Protein: 9 grams; Carbohydrates: 33 grams; Fat: 7 grams; Fiber: 6 grams

Homemade Veggie Burgers

VEGETARIAN   HIGH-FIBER

1 cup instant uncooked brown rice

1 tablespoon vegetable oil

1 onion, finely chopped

2 garlic cloves, minced

1 teaspoon thyme

1 medium carrot, peeled and grated

$\frac{1}{4}$ cup Parmesan cheese

2 tablespoons soy sauce

2 eggs or $\frac{1}{2}$ cup egg substitute

$\frac{1}{2}$ teaspoon pepper

1 cup seasoned bread crumbs

8 hamburger buns

low-fat cheese, optional

Prepare rice according to package directions. Chill in refrigerator for about 20 minutes.

Preheat broiler.

Heat oil in large skillet. Sauté onion, garlic, and thyme over medium heat until onion is tender. Transfer to a large bowl. Mix in chilled rice. Add carrot, Parmesan cheese, soy sauce, egg, pepper, and $\frac{1}{2}$ cup bread crumbs. Mix well. Form mixture into patties. Coat outside of burgers with remaining bread crumbs. Place burgers on broiler pan. Broil about 10 minutes on each side until golden brown and heated throughout.

Serve on buns with melted cheese, if desired.

Makes 8 servings
Calories: 201; Protein: 7 grams; Carbohydrates: 32 grams; Fat: 5 grams; Fiber: 3 grams

Turkey Burgers

HIGHER FAT

1 pound ground turkey

$\frac{1}{4}$ cup chopped green onions

1 clove garlic, minced

2 tablespoons rolled oats

$\frac{1}{4}$ teaspoon salt

$\frac{1}{4}$ teaspoon pepper

4 rolls or hamburger buns

In a large bowl, combine ground turkey, onion, garlic, oats, salt, and pepper. Form mixture into patties about $\frac{1}{2}$-inch thick.

Broil or grill turkey patties, turning once during cooking. Serve on rolls or buns with desired condiments.

Makes 4 servings
Calories: 304; Protein: 24 grams; Carbohydrates: 24 grams; Fat: 12 grams; Fiber: 2 grams

Greek Pasta Stir-Fry

HIGHER FAT   VEGETARIAN   HIGH-FIBER

1 cup uncooked pasta, any shape

1 tablespoon vegetable oil

½ cup fresh mushrooms, sliced

1 zucchini, thinly sliced

½ red bell pepper, chopped

1 onion, chopped

10 cherry tomatoes, sliced

10 black olives, sliced

¼ cup feta cheese

Prepare pasta according to package directions. Drain.

Heat oil in large skillet. Sauté mushrooms, zucchini, pepper, and onion until tender. Add tomatoes, olives, and cooked pasta. Heat thoroughly. Remove from heat and add feta cheese before serving.

Makes 4 servings
Calories: 206; Protein: 5 grams; Carbohydrates: 30 grams; Fat: 8 grams; Fiber: 5 grams

Spaghetti with Cherry Tomatoes

HIGHER FAT   VEGETARIAN

½ pound uncooked spaghetti

1 pint cherry tomatoes

¼ cup vegetable or olive oil

2 teaspoons chopped fresh basil

1 tablespoon margarine

¼ cup seasoned bread crumbs

2 tablespoons cup grated Parmesan cheese

Cook pasta according to package directions. Drain.

Cut cherry tomatoes into quarters. In large bowl, combine tomatoes with oil and basil. Add cooked spaghetti. Toss.

Melt margarine in medium skillet. Add bread crumbs. Toss until well coated. Remove from heat. Add Parmesan cheese. Toss well. Pour onto spaghetti mixture and toss well before serving.

Makes 6 servings
Calories: 276; Protein: 7 grams; Carbohydrates: 34 grams; Fat: 12 grams; Fiber: 2 grams

Mozzarella, Tomato, and Basil Couscous Salad

VEGETARIAN HIGH-FIBER

2 tomatoes, chopped

4 ounces part-skim mozzarella cheese, shredded

2 spring onions, chopped

1 garlic clove, minced

$\frac{1}{2}$ teaspoon salt

$\frac{1}{2}$ teaspoon pepper

2 teaspoons vegetable oil

1 cup uncooked couscous

$\frac{1}{4}$ cup chopped fresh basil

Combine tomatoes, cheese, onions, garlic, salt, and pepper in large bowl. Toss with oil. Cover and refrigerate 30 to 45 minutes.

In large saucepan, prepare couscous according to package directions. Fluff with fork. Cool.

Add vegetable-cheese mixture to couscous. Toss gently. Sprinkle with basil before serving.

Makes 6 servings
Calories: 196; Protein: 9 grams; Carbohydrates: 29 grams; Fat: 5 grams; Fiber: 3.5 grams

Pasta Alfredo

HIGHER FAT VEGETARIAN

1 pound uncooked fettuccini noodles or other pasta of choice

$\frac{1}{2}$ cup half-and-half

1 cup evaporated skim milk

1 tablespoon butter

$1\frac{1}{2}$ cups grated fresh Parmesan cheese

$\frac{1}{2}$ teaspoon pepper

1 tablespoon fresh basil

Cook pasta according to package directions. Drain and set aside.

In large saucepan, combine half-and-half, milk, and butter. Heat until butter is melted and the mixture is hot. Slowly stir in the Parmesan cheese. Cook over low heat until cheese is melted and mixture

(continued)

begins to thicken. Add pepper. Stir. Add pasta to cream mixture and toss until well coated.

Garnish with fresh basil before serving.

Makes 8 servings
Calories: 286; Protein: 14 grams; Carbohydrates: 36 grams; Fat: 10 grams; Fiber: 2 grams

Crustless Vegetable Quiche

VEGETARIAN

vegetable oil cooking spray

1 cup fresh broccoli florets

1 cup fresh cauliflower florets

$\frac{1}{2}$ cup sliced fresh mushrooms

4 eggs, beaten

$\frac{1}{2}$ cup low-fat milk

2 cups cooked rice

salt and pepper to taste

2 ounces part-skim mozzarella cheese

2 ounces low-fat Cheddar cheese

Preheat oven to 325°F. Spray 10-inch quiche pan or pie plate with cooking spray.

In medium covered saucepan, steam broccoli and cauliflower with 2 tablespoons water until softened.

In large bowl, combine mushrooms, eggs, milk, rice, salt, and pepper. Add steamed vegetables and cheeses. Stir gently.

Pour mixture into prepared pan. Bake 30 to 35 minutes or until golden brown and cooked throughout. Cool slightly before cutting and serving.

Makes 8 servings
Calories: 130; Protein: 8 grams; Carbohydrates: 15 grams; Fat: 4 grams; Fiber: 1 gram

Baked Pasta and Cheese

VEGETARIAN

$1\frac{1}{2}$ cups uncooked pasta (any shape)

1 $10\frac{3}{4}$-ounce can Cheddar cheese soup

$\frac{2}{3}$ cup low-fat milk

dash pepper

1 tablespoon seasoned bread crumbs

Prepare pasta according to package directions. Drain.

Preheat oven to 400°F.

In a 1-quart casserole dish, combine pasta with soup, milk, and pepper. Sprinkle bread crumbs over top. Bake 20 to 30 minutes or until lightly browned on top.

Makes 6 servings
Calories: 142; Protein: 7 grams; Carbohydrates: 22 grams; Fat: 4 grams; Fiber: 1 gram

Macaroni and Cheese

VEGETARIAN

1 pound uncooked elbow macaroni

1 cup low-fat milk

$\frac{1}{4}$ cup all-purpose flour

4 ounces low-fat Cheddar cheese

2 tablespoons butter

$\frac{1}{2}$ teaspoon dry mustard

$\frac{1}{2}$ teaspoon paprika

$\frac{1}{2}$ teaspoon pepper

Prepare macaroni according to package directions. Drain.

Heat milk just to hot, not to boiling.

In blender, combine flour, cheese, butter, and seasonings. Pulse to mix. Add hot milk and purée. Return drained noodles to saucepan. Add sauce. Cook over medium heat until sauce thickens.

Makes 12 servings
Calories: 187; Protein: 8 grams; Carbohydrates: 31 grams; Fat: 4 grams; Fiber: 1 gram

Spaghetti Pie

HIGHER FAT

vegetable oil cooking spray

6 ounces uncooked spaghetti

1 egg, beaten

$\frac{1}{4}$ cup grated fresh Parmesan cheese

1 teaspoon vegetable oil

$\frac{1}{3}$ cup chopped onion

1 pound lean ground beef, turkey, or vegetarian "ground beef"

$\frac{1}{4}$ cup low-fat sour cream

1 6-ounce can tomato paste

2 ounces part-skim mozzarella cheese, shredded

(continued)

Preheat oven to 350°F. Spray a casserole dish or glass pie pan with cooking spray.

Prepare spaghetti according to package directions. Drain. In a large bowl, combine warm noodles with egg and Parmesan cheese. Pour mixture into prepared pan and, using a large spoon, pat mixture around the sides and bottom of the dish.

Heat oil in large skillet. Add onion and sauté until onion is tender. Add ground meat and cook thoroughly. Drain excess fat. Add sour cream, tomato paste, and $\frac{3}{4}$ cup water. Reduce heat and simmer 10 minutes. Pour mixture into casserole dish on top of spaghetti. Bake 25 minutes. Sprinkle with mozzarella cheese. Return to oven for 1 or 2 minutes until cheese is melted.

Makes 6 servings

Calories: 383; Protein: 28 grams; Carbohydrates: 27 grams; Fat: 18 grams; Fiber: 2 grams

Vegetarian Pasta Bake

VEGETARIAN   HIGH-FIBER

1 16-ounce package uncooked pasta

1 tablespoon vegetable oil

1 onion, chopped

1 28-ounce can crushed tomatoes, undrained

1 teaspoon oregano

salt and pepper to taste

$\frac{1}{2}$ cup low-fat shredded Cheddar cheese, divided

$\frac{1}{2}$ cup part-skim mozzarella cheese, divided

Prepare pasta according to package directions. Drain. Preheat oven to 325°F.

Heat oil in large saucepan. Sauté onion for 1 minute. Add tomatoes, oregano, and salt and pepper if desired. Cook for 5 minutes until heated throughout. Stir in cooked pasta and $\frac{1}{4}$ cup each of the Cheddar and mozzarella cheeses.

Pour pasta mixture into casserole dish. Sprinkle top with remaining cheeses. Bake 20 minutes or until mixture is heated and cheese is melted.

Makes 6 servings

Calories: 330; Protein: 16 grams; Carbohydrates: 54 grams; Fat: 7 grams; Fiber: 6 grams

Broiled Pizza

VEGETARIAN

1 large pita bread

$\frac{1}{4}$ cup tomato-based pasta sauce

$\frac{1}{2}$ cup part-skim shredded mozzarella

$\frac{1}{4}$ teaspoon dried oregano

$\frac{1}{4}$ teaspoon dried basil

1 tablespoon grated Parmesan cheese

Preheat broiler.

Split pita bread in half horizontally. Broil until lightly toasted. Spread pasta sauce on each half. Sprinkle with mozzarella cheese, oregano, basil, and Parmesan cheese. Broil until cheese melts.

Makes 2 servings
Calories: 174; Protein: 10 grams; Carbohydrates: 19 grams; Fat: 6 grams; Fiber: 1.5 grams

Lots of Veggies Pizza

VEGETARIAN

1 refrigerated pizza crust (or try English muffins, tortillas, or pita bread)

1 cup tomato purée, pizza sauce, or pasta sauce

1 teaspoon oregano

2 teaspoons basil

1 teaspoon garlic powder (or fresh garlic, if preferred)

6 ounces part-skim mozzarella cheese, shredded

1 ounce grated Parmesan cheese

2 to 3 cups chopped fresh vegetables of choice (broccoli, red or green bell pepper, onions, mushrooms, zucchini, spinach, sliced tomatoes)

Preheat oven to 450°F.

Place pizza crust on cookie sheet. In small bowl, combine tomato purée or sauce with oregano, basil, and garlic. Spread over crust. Alternate layers of mozzarella cheese with vegetables, ending with cheese on top. Sprinkle with Parmesan cheese. Bake on middle shelf of oven until cheese is melted, about 10 to 12 minutes.

Makes 8 servings
Calories: 190; Protein: 11 grams; Carbohydrates: 24 grams; Fat: 6 grams; Fiber: 2 grams

Fresh Tomato Pizza

VEGETARIAN

1 large packaged pizza crust or refrigerated pizza crust

1 tablespoon vegetable oil

4 plum tomatoes, thinly sliced

$\frac{1}{2}$ cup shredded part-skim mozzarella cheese

$\frac{1}{4}$ cup fresh basil, chopped

3 garlic cloves, minced

$\frac{1}{2}$ teaspoon salt

$\frac{1}{2}$ teaspoon pepper

Preheat oven to 400°F or as directed on pizza crust package.

Drizzle oil over crust. Layer tomatoes, cheese, basil, and garlic over crust. Sprinkle with salt and pepper. For extra fiber, top with chopped vegetables, if desired.

Bake 5 to 10 minutes until crust is hot and cheese is melted.

Makes 8 servings
Calories: 133; Protein: 5 grams; Carbohydrates: 18 grams; Fat: 4 grams; Fiber: 1 gram

Ratatouille

HIGHER FAT   VEGETARIAN   HIGH-FIBER

$\frac{1}{4}$ cup vegetable oil

2 garlic cloves, minced

$\frac{1}{2}$ teaspoon salt

$\frac{1}{2}$ teaspoon dried rosemary, crushed

$\frac{1}{4}$ teaspoon black pepper

1 small eggplant, peeled and thinly sliced

3 plum tomatoes, thinly sliced

3 small zucchini, thinly sliced

4 new potatoes, thinly sliced

Preheat oven to 425°F.

In small bowl, combine oil, garlic, salt, rosemary, and pepper. Set aside.

In round casserole dish, layer vegetables in a pattern: first $\frac{1}{3}$ of the eggplant, then $\frac{1}{3}$ of the tomatoes, $\frac{1}{3}$ of the zucchini, and $\frac{1}{3}$ of the potatoes; continue until all the vegetables are used. Overlap each slice when layering. Drizzle oil-spice mixture over the vegetables.

Cover and bake 15 minutes. Uncover and bake an additional 30 to 35 minutes or until vegetables are tender and browned.

Makes 6 servings
Calories: 198; Protein: 4 grams; Carbohydrates: 27 grams; Fat: 9 grams; Fiber: 5 grams

Chicken and Pasta with Peanut Sauce

HIGH-FIBER

2 boneless, skinless chicken breasts

teriyaki or soy sauce, to taste

$\frac{3}{4}$ cup uncooked pasta, any shape

$\frac{1}{2}$ cup frozen peas

2 carrots, sliced in circles

$\frac{1}{2}$ cup broccoli, chopped

2 tablespoons creamy peanut butter

2 tablespoons low-fat milk

1 tablespoon soy sauce

1 tablespoon lime juice

cayenne pepper to taste

Brush chicken with teriyaki or soy sauce. Grill, broil, or microwave until chicken is thoroughly cooked and no longer pink inside.

Cook pasta in boiling water until just tender, 3 or 4 minutes. Add peas, carrots, and broccoli, cooking an additional 3 or 4 minutes.

In separate small saucepan, warm the peanut butter. Add milk and blend with a fork. Add soy sauce, lime juice, and a dash of cayenne pepper. Add more milk for a thinner sauce.

Drain pasta mixture and put on serving plate. Cut hot chicken into strips and place on top of pasta. Pour peanut sauce over pasta and chicken before serving.

Makes 4 servings
Calories: 265; Protein: 33 grams; Carbohydrates: 19 grams; Fat: 6 grams; Fiber: 3.5 grams

Tuna and Cheese Pocket Melts

2 6-ounce cans water-packed tuna, drained

2 tablespoons low-fat mayonnaise

3 pita breads

4 ounces shredded cheese (part-skim mozzarella, low-fat American, or
    Cheddar)

Preheat oven or toaster oven to 350°F.

In small bowl, combine tuna with mayonnaise. Cut pita breads in half, making 2 half-round pockets from each pita. Stuff each half with about ¼ cup of the tuna mixture. Top tuna with cheese. Place on cookie sheet and bake 10 to 15 minutes or until cheese is melted.

Makes 6 servings
Calories: 216; Protein: 22 grams; Carbohydrates: 18 grams; Fat: 6 grams; Fiber: 1 gram

Cashew Chicken Casserole

HIGHER FAT

4 boneless, skinless chicken breasts, cut into cubes

1 medium onion, diced

3 chicken bouillon cubes

8 ounces sliced fresh mushrooms (or a 10-ounce can)

1 cup uncooked long-grain rice

2 teaspoons powdered ginger

1½ cups boiling water

2 cups chopped broccoli

½ cup cashew nuts

salt, pepper, garlic, and soy sauce to taste

Preheat oven to 375°F.

In 2-quart casserole, combine chicken, onion, and one crushed bouillon cube. Cover and microwave on medium heat for 5 minutes, stirring once.

Add mushrooms, rice, ginger, boiling water, and remaining bouillon cubes to casserole dish. Cover and bake 30 minutes. Add broccoli, cover, and cook an additional 10 minutes. Allow dish to stand for several minutes. Add half of the cashews, salt, pepper, garlic, and soy sauce, as desired. Stir. Add remaining cashews on top and broil (without cover) to brown top.

Makes 6 servings
Calories: 331; Protein: 42 grams; Carbohydrates: 23 grams; Fat: 8 grams; Fiber: 2 grams

Chicken Scallopini

HIGHER FAT

4 boneless, skinless chicken breasts

¼ cup bread crumbs

¼ cup grated Parmesan cheese

2 tablespoons vegetable oil

2 tablespoons lemon juice

Place chicken breasts between two pieces of wax paper and flatten with a mallet to about ½-inch thick.

Combine bread crumbs and Parmesan cheese in pie pan or plate. Coat each chicken breast with breadcrumb mixture.

Heat oil in large skillet over medium heat. Brown chicken breasts, about 3 to 5 minutes on each side, until chicken is no longer pink. Transfer chicken breasts to platter. Add lemon juice to drippings in pan. Turn heat to high and stir while scraping the browned crumbs into the sauce. Pour sauce over chicken. Serve immediately.

Makes 4 servings

Calories: 242; Protein: 30 grams; Carbohydrates: 6 grams; Fat: 11 grams; Fiber: none

Skillet Barbecue

1 small onion, sliced

1 teaspoon olive or vegetable oil

½ pound skinless and boneless chicken breasts, turkey cutlets, or cubed
  steak

¼ cup barbecue sauce

Heat oil in a 9-inch skillet and sauté onion over low heat, until tender. Increase heat to medium and push the onions to one side. Add chicken to skillet. Cook 3 to 4 minutes. Turn chicken over and brush with barbecue sauce. Continue to cook an additional 5 minutes or until done. Serve with the onions.

Makes 2 servings

Calories: 182; Protein: 28 grams; Carbohydrates: 7 grams; Fat: 4 grams; Fiber: 1 gram

Old Fashioned Beef Stew

HIGHER FAT   HIGH-FIBER

1 pound beef cubes, well trimmed

½ cup all-purpose flour

2 tablespoons vegetable oil

½ teaspoon garlic salt

½ teaspoon onion salt

½ teaspoon pepper

1 onion, cut into wedges

3 carrots, sliced

2 celery stalks, sliced

1 10½-ounce can condensed beef broth

4 potatoes, cut into wedges

In large bowl, toss beef cubes with flour. Heat oil in large Dutch oven or pot. Add beef and seasonings. Sauté for about 5 minutes until beef is browned.

Add onion, carrots, celery, and broth. Cover and reduce heat. Simmer for 45 minutes or until vegetables are tender. Add potatoes. Cover and simmer another 20 minutes until potatoes are tender and soft. Serve immediately.

Makes 6 servings

Calories: 334; Protein: 23 grams; Carbohydrates: 34 grams; Fat: 12 grams; Fiber: 4 grams

Easy Baked Fish Fillets

1 pound fish fillets—scrod, sole, or other similar fish

½ cup cornmeal

1 teaspoon dried parsley

1 teaspoon minced onion

1 teaspoon garlic salt

1 teaspoon dried basil

dash pepper

1 tablespoon vegetable oil

Combine cornmeal, parsley, onion, garlic salt, basil, and pepper in a pie pan or shallow dish. Dip fish fillets into cornmeal mixture. Coat on both sides.

Heat oil in large skillet over medium heat. Cook each fish fillet 4 to 5 minutes until browned on each side and fish flakes easily with a fork.

Remove from heat. Serve immediately.

Makes 4 servings
Calories: 190; Protein: 23 grams; Carbohydrates: 12 grams; Fat: 5 grams; Fiber: 1 gram

SENSATIONAL SIDES

Crispy Hash Browns

VEGETARIAN   HIGH-FIBER

2 tablespoons vegetable oil
4 large white potatoes, sliced thin or shredded
1 large onion, chopped
$\frac{1}{2}$ teaspoon garlic powder
salt and pepper to taste

Heat oil in skillet over medium-high heat. Add potatoes, onion, garlic powder, salt, and pepper. Stir-fry until potatoes become crispy, about 15 minutes.

Makes 4 servings
Calories: 279; Protein: 5 grams; Carbohydrates: 51 grams; Fat: 7 grams; Fiber: 5 grams

Awesome Potato Skins

VEGETARIAN

2 potatoes
salt and pepper to taste
2 tablespoons heart-healthy margarine
$\frac{1}{2}$ cup low-fat cheese
$\frac{1}{4}$ cup low-fat plain yogurt or sour cream, optional
optional add-ins: bacon bits, olives, guacamole, cottage cheese

Preheat oven to 400°F.

Wash potatoes, prick with a fork, and bake for 1 hour. Leave oven on. When cool enough to handle, cut potatoes in half lengthwise, then cut again lengthwise. Scoop out insides, leaving $\frac{1}{4}$-inch of cooked potato in skin. (Save the cooked potato you remove for another recipe or for Smashed Mashed Potatoes.)

Arrange skins in an oven-proof dish and sprinkle with salt and pepper (and other seasonings, if desired). Spread margarine on skins, then sprinkle with cheese. Return to oven for 5 to 10 minutes until cheese melts.

(continued)

Top with yogurt and other add-ins if desired.

Makes 4 servings
Calories: 120; Protein: 5 grams; Carbohydrates: 16 grams; Fat: 4 grams; Fiber: 1 gram

Smashed Mashed Potatoes

LOWER FAT   VEGETARIAN   HIGH-FIBER

2 baking or red potatoes, or leftover baked potato flesh from Awesome
    Potato Skins
2 teaspoons heart-healthy margarine
$\frac{1}{4}$ cup 1% milk or skim milk
salt, pepper, garlic, or other seasonings, as desired

Peel potatoes, if desired. Cut potatoes into quarters and put in
medium saucepan with enough water to cover them. Bring to boil and
cook for 20 minutes, or until soft. Drain. Put potatoes into a large bowl
for mashing. (You can also use a food processor.) Add margarine and
milk. Mash or blend until smooth. (Do not overblend.) Add salt, pepper, or other seasonings to taste.

If using leftover potato from Awesome Potato Skins, mash or
blend potatoes as directed.

Makes 2 servings
Calories: 164; Protein: 4 grams; Carbohydrates: 32 grams; Fat: 2 grams; Fiber: 3 grams

Sweet Potato Fries

LOWER FAT   VEGETARIAN   HIGH-FIBER

2 large sweet potatoes, peeled and cut lengthwise into thin wedges
$\frac{1}{2}$ teaspoon salt
dash chili powder
dash pepper
vegetable oil cooking spray

Preheat oven to 425°F.

Place potato wedges and seasonings in a resealable plastic bag.
Shake until well coated.

Place potato wedges on cookie sheet coated with cooking spray.
Spray tops of potato wedges with cooking spray.

Bake 10 minutes. Turn potatoes over to keep from sticking. Bake
an additional 10 minutes until crispy and browned.

Makes 2 servings
Calories: 137; Protein: 2 grams; Carbohydrates: 32 grams; Fat: 0; Fiber: 4 grams

Carrot Soufflé

VEGETARIAN

1 pound carrots

4 tablespoons margarine, melted

3 eggs

$\frac{1}{2}$ cup sugar

3 tablespoons all-purpose flour

1 teaspoon baking powder

1 teaspoon vanilla extract

dash salt

vegetable oil cooking spray

Preheat oven to 275°F.

Peel carrots and cut into large slices. In large saucepan, cook carrots in water until soft. Drain.

Combine remaining ingredients in food processor or blender. Add carrots and blend well until mixture is smooth. Add salt, if desired.

Pour mixture into a casserole dish coated with cooking spray. Bake 45 minutes or until firm.

Makes 10 servings
Calories: 128; Protein: 3 grams; Carbohydrates: 17 grams; Fat: 6 grams; Fiber: 1 gram

Pumpkin Casserole

VEGETARIAN

1 15-ounce can pumpkin

4 tablespoons margarine

1 cup sugar

1 cup all-purpose flour

4 eggs

$\frac{1}{4}$ cup low-fat milk

vegetable oil cooking spray

$\frac{1}{2}$ teaspoon cinnamon

Preheat oven to 350°F.

In large saucepan, cook pumpkin and margarine together over low heat. When margarine has melted, remove from heat and pour into a large mixing bowl. Beat sugar and flour into pumpkin mixture.

(continued)

In small bowl, beat eggs. Add milk. Fold into pumpkin mixture. Pour into 8-inch-square pan sprayed with cooking spray. Sprinkle cinnamon over top. Bake 45 minutes or until firm.

Cut into 2-inch squares to serve.

Makes 16 servings
Calories: 129; Protein: 3 grams; Carbohydrates: 21 grams; Fat: 4 grams; Fiber: 1.5 grams

Chinese Rice

HIGHER FAT   VEGETARIAN

$\frac{1}{3}$ cup vegetable oil

1 small onion, chopped

$\frac{1}{3}$ cup chopped fresh green onion tops

optional vegetables: $\frac{1}{4}$ to $\frac{1}{3}$ cup chopped mushrooms, zucchini, broccoli, or spinach

3 eggs

2 cups cooked rice

1 teaspoon salt

$\frac{1}{2}$ teaspoon pepper

1 14-ounce can bean sprouts, drained

soy sauce to taste

Heat oil in large skillet. Sauté onion, green onion tops, and any other vegetables you may wish to add. Beat eggs in small bowl, then add to skillet. Cook several minutes, breaking up the egg mixture with a fork while cooking. Add rice, salt, pepper, and sprouts. Sprinkle with soy sauce while cooking. Cook 10 minutes, just until hot. Cover pan for several minutes to heat thoroughly. If too dry, add additional soy sauce or oil. Toss with two forks before serving. Leftover chicken may be added to rice to make a main dish.

Makes 8 servings
Calories: 176; Protein: 4 grams; Carbohydrates: 16 grams; Fat: 11 grams; Fiber: 1 gram

Noodles with Peanut Sauce

HIGHER FAT   VEGETARIAN   HIGH-FIBER

4 ounces uncooked spaghetti

$\frac{1}{4}$ cup peanut butter

$\frac{1}{2}$ cup boiling water

$\frac{1}{4}$ cup soy sauce

2 teaspoons honey

1 garlic clove, crushed

$\frac{1}{2}$ teaspoon powdered ginger

3 green onions, chopped

1 14-ounce can bean sprouts, drained

$\frac{1}{4}$ cup chopped peanuts

Prepare pasta according to package directions. Drain.

Put peanut butter in large bowl. Add boiling water and whisk until smooth. Add soy sauce, honey, garlic, and ginger. Whisk again until smooth.

Add cooked noodles, green onions, bean sprouts, and peanuts to peanut butter mixture. Toss well. Serve immediately.

Makes 4 servings
Calories: 289; Protein: 14 grams; Carbohydrates: 32 grams; Fat: 13 grams; Fiber: 4 grams

Noodle Kugel

VEGETARIAN

vegetable oil cooking spray

8 ounces wide noodles

3 eggs

1 cup low-fat sour cream

1 cup low-fat cottage cheese

$\frac{1}{2}$ cup brown sugar

$\frac{3}{4}$ cup raisins

1 cup orange juice

1 apple, peeled and sliced thin, optional

$\frac{1}{4}$ cup dry cereal

1 tablespoon margarine

Preheat oven to 350°F. Spray 8-by-8-inch casserole with cooking spray.

Cook noodles in 6 cups boiling water about 8 to 9 minutes or until tender. Drain.

In a large bowl, beat eggs slightly. Add sour cream, cottage cheese, brown sugar, raisins, orange juice, and apple (if using). Add noodles and mix well. Pour mixture into prepared pan. Crush cereal and place on top of casserole before baking. Dot with small amounts of margarine. Bake $1\frac{1}{2}$ hours or until bubbling and browned.

Makes 16 servings
Calories: 168; Protein: 6 grams; Carbohydrates: 28 grams; Fat: 4 grams; Fiber: 1 gram

Crunchy Chicken Salad

1 cup cubed cooked chicken

1 stalk celery, chopped

½ cup diced apple

½ cup sliced grapes

2 tablespoons low-fat mayonnaise

½ teaspoon celery salt

Combine all ingredients in medium bowl. Serve on a roll or bun, stuffed in a tomato, or over lettuce.

Makes 2 servings
Calories: 197; Protein: 20 grams; Carbohydrates: 16 grams; Fat: 6 grams; Fiber: 1 gram

Spinach Fruit Salad

HIGHER FAT   VEGETARIAN

Dressing:

¾ cup raspberry vinegar

¼ cup vegetable oil

½ cup sugar

2 tablespoons finely chopped red onion

¼ teaspoon garlic powder

¼ teaspoon salt

1 to 2 tablespoons poppy seeds

Salad:

1 pound spinach, cleaned and stemmed

1 16-ounce can mandarin oranges, drained, or 1 cup sliced fresh strawberries

½ pound mushrooms sliced

½ red onion, sliced

¼ cup sunflower seeds, or 2 tablespoons sesame seeds

Combine dressing ingredients. Refrigerate for up to 24 hours. Combine salad ingredients. Pour dressing over salad. Serve immediately.

Makes 8 servings
Calories: 188; Protein: 4 grams; Carbohydrates: 27 grams; Fat: 9 grams; Fiber: 2 grams

Warm Pasta and Spinach Salad

VEGETARIAN   HIGH-FIBER

8 ounces uncooked bowtie pasta

1 tablespoon vegetable oil

3 garlic cloves, minced

$1\frac{1}{2}$ cup red bell pepper, chopped

1 cup sliced mushrooms

1 zucchini, thinly sliced

10 green olives, sliced

3 tablespoons balsamic vinegar

1 tablespoon spicy brown mustard

6 cups fresh spinach leaves, torn into bite-sized pieces

$\frac{1}{4}$ cup finely grated Parmesan cheese

Cook pasta according to package directions. Drain.

In large skillet, heat oil over medium heat. Sauté garlic, bell pepper, mushrooms, zucchini, and olives until tender.

In large bowl, combine drained pasta with the vegetable mixture. In small bowl, combine vinegar with mustard. Toss with pasta and vegetables. Add spinach. Toss again. Top with Parmesan cheese. Serve immediately.

Makes 4 servings
Calories: 191; Protein: 8 grams; Carbohydrates: 25 grams; Fat: 7 grams; Fiber: 4 grams

Veggie Pasta Casserole

LOWER FAT   VEGETARIAN

1 cup fresh cauliflower florets

1 cup fresh broccoli florets

4 ounces uncooked pasta, any shape

$\frac{1}{4}$ cup all-purpose flour

1 cup low-fat milk

$\frac{1}{4}$ teaspoon thyme

1 garlic clove, minced

$\frac{1}{2}$ cup shredded sharp Cheddar cheese

$\frac{1}{4}$ cup grated Parmesan cheese

2 spring onions, chopped

2 teaspoons spicy mustard

dash pepper

$\frac{1}{2}$ cup seasoned bread crumbs

(continued)

Preheat oven to 400°F.

Cook cauliflower and broccoli in 4 cups boiling water until tender. Remove vegetables, reserve water. Cook pasta in reserved water until tender. Drain.

Heat flour, milk, thyme, and garlic in large saucepan, stirring constantly, until mixture begins to thicken. Remove from heat. Add Cheddar and Parmesan cheeses, onions, mustard, and pepper. Add vegetables and pasta. Spoon mixture into 9-by-13-inch baking pan. Top with bread crumbs. Bake 20 to 25 minutes until lightly browned and cooked through.

Makes 12 servings

Calories: 100; Protein: 6 grams; Carbohydrates: 15 grams; Fat: 2 grams; Fiber: 1 gram

Broccoli and Rice Bake

VEGETARIAN

vegetable oil cooking spray

1 bunch broccoli, trimmed and cut into $\frac{3}{4}$-inch pieces (about 2 cups)

1 tablespoon vegetable oil

1 teaspoon salt

2 cups uncooked white rice

$3\frac{1}{2}$ cups water

1 egg, beaten

dash paprika

Preheat oven to 375°F. Spray 2-quart casserole with cooking spray.

In large saucepan, combine broccoli, oil, salt, rice, and water. Cook on medium to high heat 15 to 20 minutes, until water is absorbed. Add beaten egg and mix thoroughly. Pour mixture into prepared casserole dish. Sprinkle paprika on top. Bake 45 minutes or until lightly browned on top.

Makes 6 servings

Calories: 265; Protein: 6 grams; Carbohydrates: 51 grams; Fat: 4 grams; Fiber: 2 grams

Vegetable Stir-Fry with a Twist

VEGETARIAN   HIGH-FIBER

$1\frac{1}{2}$ tablespoons vegetable oil

1 medium onion, cut into rings

6 baby corns, cut into small pieces

$\frac{1}{2}$ cup thinly sliced carrots

1 cup chopped broccoli

$\frac{3}{4}$ cup bean sprouts

$\frac{1}{2}$ small red bell pepper, cut into strips

1 small zucchini, cut into thin circles

1 8-ounce can bamboo shoots

1 8-ounce can sliced water chestnuts

garlic, pepper, and salt to taste

Sauce:

5 ounces vegetable broth

$\frac{1}{2}$ tablespoon cornstarch mixed with 1 tablespoon warm water

2 teaspoons brown sugar

1 tablespoon soy sauce

Heat oil in large skillet. Add onion and cook until softened, about 5 minutes. Add remaining vegetables and seasonings. Stir-fry until all vegetables are tender.

Make sauce. In small saucepan, combine vegetable broth with cornstarch paste. Heat over low heat. Add brown sugar and soy sauce. Turn heat to high and bring to a boil. Reduce heat and simmer about 2 minutes until sauce thickens. Pour sauce over hot vegetables and toss.

Makes 6 servings
Calories: 108; Protein: 3 grams; Carbohydrates: 18 grams; Fat: 4 grams; Fiber: 4 grams

Vegetable Chow Mein

LOWER FAT   VEGETARIAN   HIGH-FIBER

1 tablespoon vegetable oil

$\frac{1}{2}$ cup vegetable broth

3 cups cooked rice

1 cup bean sprouts, fresh or canned, drained

1 stalk celery, chopped

1 large red bell pepper, seeded and chopped

1 large carrot, chopped

8 ounces sliced mushrooms

soy sauce to taste

In large skillet, heat oil and broth. Sauté rice and vegetables over medium heat for about 15 minutes until thoroughly cooked. Stir frequently. Add soy sauce to taste.

Makes 6 servings
Calories: 173; Protein: 5 grams; Carbohydrates: 32 grams; Fat: 3 grams; Fiber: 3 grams

Parmesan Couscous

VEGETARIAN

1 tablespoon vegetable oil

$\frac{1}{4}$ cup chopped onion

2 cloves garlic, minced

1 cup uncooked couscous

1 14$\frac{1}{2}$-ounce can chicken broth

$\frac{1}{2}$ cup Parmesan cheese

$\frac{1}{2}$ teaspoon salt

$\frac{1}{2}$ teaspoon pepper

Heat oil in large skillet. Add onion and garlic and sauté until tender. Add couscous and chicken broth. Cook, covered, for 5 minutes. Fluff couscous with fork. Add Parmesan cheese, salt, and pepper. Fluff again. Serve immediately.

Makes 6 servings
Calories: 192; Protein: 11 grams; Carbohydrates: 23 grams; Fat: 6 grams; Fiber: 2 grams

BAKED BEAUTIES

Peanut Butter and Chocolate Chip Snackers

VEGETARIAN

vegetable oil cooking spray

1 cup all-purpose flour

$\frac{1}{2}$ cup sugar

$\frac{1}{4}$ cup brown sugar

1 teaspoon baking powder

dash salt

$\frac{1}{2}$ cup low-fat milk

$\frac{1}{3}$ cup creamy peanut butter

2 tablespoons softened margarine

1 teaspoon vanilla extract

1 egg

$\frac{1}{3}$ cup semisweet chocolate chips

Preheat oven to 350°F. Spray muffin tin with cooking spray or line with paper baking cups.

In large mixing bowl, combine all ingredients except chocolate chips. Mix until smooth. Blend in chocolate chips. Spoon batter into prepared pan, filling each cup $\frac{2}{3}$ full. Bake 18 to 20 minutes or until lightly browned and toothpick inserted comes out clean. Remove from oven. Cool.

Makes 1 dozen
Calories: 175; Protein: 4 grams; Carbohydrates: 24 grams; Fat: 7 grams; Fiber: 1 gram

Banana Cake

VEGETARIAN

vegetable oil cooking spray

2 cups all-purpose flour

$1\frac{1}{2}$ cups sugar

$1\frac{1}{2}$ teaspoons baking powder

$\frac{1}{2}$ teaspoon baking soda

$\frac{1}{2}$ teaspoon salt

2 ripe bananas, mashed

$\frac{1}{2}$ cup low-fat milk

$\frac{1}{2}$ cup vegetable oil

2 eggs

1 teaspoon vanilla extract

Topping:

1 ripe banana, mashed

$\frac{1}{2}$ teaspoon lemon juice

$\frac{1}{4}$ cup softened margarine

1-pound box confectioners' sugar

Preheat oven to 350°F. Spray a 9-by-13-inch baking pan with cooking spray.

In a large bowl, combine flour, sugar, baking powder, baking soda, and salt. Add mashed bananas, milk, oil, eggs, and vanilla. Mix until well combined. Pour batter into prepared pan. Bake 25 to 30 minutes or until toothpick inserted comes out clean. Cool.

Prepare topping: Combine mashed banana, lemon juice, margarine, and confectioners' sugar.

Spread on cooled cake.

Makes 24 servings
Calories: 242; Protein: 2 grams; Carbohydrates: 43 grams; Fat: 7 grams; Fiber: .5 gram

Fruit and Cake Trifle

VEGETARIAN

1 package chocolate cake mix

2 large bananas, sliced

1 cup fresh raspberries or blueberries

2 cups prepared low-fat vanilla pudding

2 to 3 cups nonfat or low-fat whipped topping

$\frac{1}{4}$ cup toasted slivered almonds

Bake cake in 9-by-13-inch pan according to package directions. Cool. Cut cake in half crosswise. Put half away to use for another dessert. Cut remaining half into 8 pieces, then split each in half horizontally. Arrange half of the cake pieces in a 2-quart glass serving bowl.

Layer half of the bananas and berries over cake. Spread 1 cup of the pudding on top of the fruit. Repeat with remaining cake pieces, banana, berries, and pudding. Cover and chill. Top with whipped topping and sprinkle with almonds.

Variations: Use one 16-ounce package frozen strawberries or 1 pint fresh strawberries instead of bananas, and yellow or white cake instead of chocolate.

Makes 8 to 10 servings
Calories: 212; Protein: 3 grams; Carbohydrates: 41 grams; Fat: 4 grams; Fiber: 2 grams

Peanut Butter Brownies

VEGETARIAN

vegetable oil cooking spray

1 cup all-purpose flour

$\frac{1}{4}$ teaspoon baking soda

dash salt

$\frac{3}{4}$ cup sugar

$\frac{1}{4}$ cup brown sugar

$\frac{1}{4}$ cup creamy peanut butter

1 tablespoon vegetable oil

1 teaspoon vanilla extract

2 eggs

Preheat oven to 350°F. Spray 8-inch square baking pan with cooking spray.

In small bowl, combine flour, baking soda, and salt. In large mixing bowl, combine sugars, peanut butter, oil, vanilla, and eggs. Add flour mixture, mixing until just blended.

Pour batter into prepared baking pan. Bake 20 to 25 minutes or until toothpick inserted comes out clean.

Makes 16 brownies
Calories: 119; Protein: 3 grams; Carbohydrates: 20 grams; Fat: 4 grams; Fiber: none

Apple Cake

HIGHER FAT   VEGETARIAN

vegetable oil cooking spray

$\frac{1}{2}$ cup margarine

$\frac{1}{2}$ cup sugar

$\frac{1}{2}$ cup applesauce

2 eggs

1 teaspoon vanilla extract

2 cups all-purpose flour

1 teaspoon baking soda

1 teaspoon baking powder

1 cup light sour cream

Filling and Topping:

$\frac{1}{2}$ cup brown sugar

$\frac{1}{4}$ cup chopped nuts

$\frac{1}{4}$ cup sugar

1 teaspoon cinnamon

2 tart apples, peeled and sliced

Preheat oven to 325°F.

Spray a 12-cup Bundt pan with cooking spray.

Using an electric mixer, cream margarine and sugar in large bowl. Add applesauce, eggs, and vanilla. Add flour, baking soda, baking powder, and sour cream. Mix well.

Put half of the batter in prepared Bundt pan. In a small bowl, combine brown sugar, nuts, sugar, and cinnamon. Place half of the filling/topping mixture and all of the peeled apples on top of the batter. Add remaining batter and top with the remaining topping mixture. Bake 60 to 70 minutes or until a toothpick inserted comes out clean.

Makes 16 servings
Calories: 234; Protein: 4 grams; Carbohydrates: 33 grams; Fat: 10 grams; Fiber: .5 gram

Raspberry Yogurt Pie

HIGHER FAT   VEGETARIAN

1 8-ounce carton low-fat raspberry yogurt
1 8-ounce container fat-free, nondairy whipped topping, thawed
1 9-inch prepared graham cracker pie crust
$\frac{1}{2}$ cup fresh raspberries

In a large bowl, fold the yogurt into the whipped topping. Pour mixture into pie crust. Top with fresh raspberries. Refrigerate at least 2 hours before serving.

Makes 8 servings
Calories: 230; Protein: 1 grams; Carbohydrates: 36 grams; Fat: 8 grams; Fiber: 1 gram

Oatmeal Raisin Cookies

LOWER FAT   VEGETARIAN

vegetable oil cooking spray
3 cups quick-cooking oats
2 cups brown sugar, firmly packed
$\frac{1}{2}$ cup softened margarine
$\frac{1}{2}$ cup unsweetened applesauce, not chunky
2 eggs
1 teaspoon baking soda
2 teaspoons vanilla extract
$\frac{1}{2}$ teaspoon salt
2 cups all-purpose flour
$\frac{1}{2}$ cup raisins

Preheat oven to 375°F. Spray cookie sheet with cooking spray.

In large mixing bowl, combine all ingredients except flour and raisins. Beat at low speed until well mixed. Add flour and raisins. Mix together.

Drop dough by tablespoonfuls onto prepared cookie sheet, keeping 1 to 2 inches between each cookie. Bake 8 to 10 minutes or until lightly browned.

Remove cookies with spatula and place on rack to cool.

Makes 4 dozen cookies
Calories: 100; Protein: 2 grams; Carbohydrates: 18 grams; Fat: 2 grams; Fiber: 1 gram

Low-fat Chocolate Chip Cookies

LOWER FAT   VEGETARIAN

$2\frac{1}{2}$ cups all-purpose flour

$\frac{1}{2}$ cup unsweetened cocoa powder

1 teaspoon baking soda

$\frac{1}{2}$ teaspoon salt

1 teaspoon brown sugar

$\frac{3}{4}$ cup sugar

$\frac{1}{3}$ cup vegetable oil

$\frac{1}{2}$ cup unsweetened applesauce, not chunky

3 egg whites

2 teaspoons vanilla extract

$\frac{1}{2}$ cup semisweet chocolate chips

Preheat oven to 300°F.

In medium bowl, combine flour, cocoa powder, baking soda, and salt.

In another bowl, mix together the brown and white sugars, then add oil, applesauce, egg whites, and vanilla. Add flour mixture and mix until just combined. Refrigerate dough at least one hour. Roll chilled dough into 1-inch balls. Place 1 to 2 inches apart on ungreased cookie sheet and flatten slightly in the middle with your thumb. Place several chocolate chips in the center of each cookie. Bake 15 to 18 minutes or until lightly browned. (Cookies will be soft when removed from the oven, but will harden as they cool.) Remove cookies with spatula and place on rack to cool.

Makes 6 dozen cookies
Calories: 42; Protein: 1 gram; Carbohydrates: 7 grams; Fat: 1 gram; Fiber: none

Oatmeal Chocolate Chip Cookies

LOWER FAT   VEGETARIAN

2 cups brown sugar

$\frac{1}{2}$ cup margarine, softened

1 egg

$1\frac{1}{2}$ cups all-purpose flour

$\frac{3}{4}$ teaspoon baking soda

$\frac{1}{4}$ teaspoon salt

$\frac{1}{2}$ cup graham cracker crumbs

(continued)

1 cup rolled oats

½ cup semisweet chocolate chips

Preheat oven to 350°F.

In large bowl, mix together brown sugar, margarine, and egg. Add remaining ingredients. Mix well.

Drop batter by tablespoonfuls onto ungreased cookie sheet, 1 to 2 inches apart. Bake 10 minutes or until edges are lightly browned. Remove cookies with spatula and place on rack to cool.

Makes 3 ½ dozen cookies

Calories: 100; Protein: 1 gram; Carbohydrates: 17 grams; Fat: .3 grams; Fiber: 1 gram

Banana Chocolate Chip Bars

VEGETARIAN

vegetable oil cooking spray

1 cup all-purpose flour

¼ cup wheat germ

¼ teaspoon cinnamon

dash nutmeg

½ teaspoon baking powder

½ teaspoon salt

1 cup brown sugar

½ cup margarine, melted

1 egg

2 ripe bananas, mashed

1 teaspoon vanilla extract

½ cup chopped nuts

½ cup semisweet chocolate chips

Preheat oven to 350°F. Spray 9-by-13-inch baking pan with cooking spray.

In large bowl, combine flour, wheat germ, cinnamon, nutmeg, baking powder, and salt. In another bowl, combine brown sugar, margarine, egg, mashed bananas, and vanilla. Fold mixtures together until just mixed.

Pour batter into prepared baking pan. Top with chopped nuts and chocolate chips. Bake 20 to 25 minutes or until toothpick inserted comes out clean. Cool before cutting and serving.

Makes 2 dozen bars

Calories: 136; Protein: 2 grams; Carbohydrates: 19 grams; Fat: 7 grams; Fiber: 1 gram

Apple Walnut Cookies

VEGETARIAN

$1\frac{1}{2}$ cups rolled oats

$\frac{1}{2}$ teaspoon allspice

4 tablespoons margarine

3 tablespoons brown sugar

1 apple, peeled, cored, and chopped

$\frac{1}{4}$ cup chopped walnuts

1 egg

Preheat oven to 400°F.

In medium bowl, combine oats, allspice, and margarine. Mix well. Add remaining ingredients.

Mix until well combined.

Roll batter into balls and arrange on nonstick cookie sheet. Flatten slightly with spatula. Bake 10 minutes or until lightly browned. Remove cookies with spatula and place on rack to cool.

Makes 1 dozen cookies
Calories: 100; Protein: 2 grams; Carbohydrates: 10 grams; Fat: 6 grams; Fiber: 1 gram

Lemon Glazed Zucchini Bread

VEGETARIAN

vegetable oil cooking spray

$2\frac{1}{2}$ cups all-purpose flour

$\frac{3}{4}$ cup sugar

1 teaspoon baking powder

$\frac{1}{2}$ teaspoon baking soda

1 teaspoon cinnamon

dash nutmeg

$\frac{1}{2}$ teaspoon salt

1 cup finely shredded zucchini

$\frac{1}{2}$ cup low-fat milk

$\frac{1}{4}$ cup vegetable oil

2 tablespoons lemon juice

1 egg

Glaze:

1 cup confectioners' sugar

2 tablespoons lemon juice

(continued)

Preheat oven to 350°F. Spray a 9-by-5-by-3-inch loaf pan with cooking spray.

In large bowl, combine flour, sugar, baking powder, baking soda, cinnamon, nutmeg, and salt. In a small bowl, combine zucchini, milk, oil, lemon juice, and egg. Make a well in the center of the flour mixture. Add liquid mixture and fold together until just moist.

Spoon batter into prepared loaf pan. Bake 1 hour or until toothpick inserted comes out clean. Cool 10 minutes before removing from pan.

Combine glaze ingredients. Drizzle over cooled bread.

Makes 1 loaf or 12 servings
Calories: 240; Protein: 4 grams; Carbohydrates: 44 grams; Fat: 5 grams; Fiber: none

Quick and Easy Zucchini Loaf

HIGHER FAT   VEGETARIAN

vegetable oil cooking spray

2 eggs

1 cup sugar

½ cup vegetable oil

1 teaspoon vanilla extract

1½ cups all-purpose flour

1 teaspoon baking soda

½ teaspoon cinnamon

¼ teaspoon nutmeg

1 cup shredded or finely chopped zucchini (about 2 medium)

Preheat oven to 350°F. Spray 9-by-5-by-3-inch loaf pan with cooking spray.

In large mixing bowl, beat together eggs, sugar, oil, and vanilla. Add flour, baking soda, cinnamon, and nutmeg. Fold in zucchini.

Pour batter into prepared loaf pan. Bake 50 to 60 minutes or until toothpick inserted comes out clean.

Makes 1 loaf or 12 servings
Calories: 218; Protein: 3 grams; Carbohydrates: 30 grams; Fat: 10 grams; Fiber: none

Baked Apples

LOWER FAT   VEGETARIAN   HIGH-FIBER

¾ cup brown sugar

1 cup water

1 tablespoon margarine

½ teaspoon cinnamon

dash nutmeg

4 large tart baking apples

Preheat oven to 350°F.

In saucepan over medium heat, combine brown sugar, water, margarine, cinnamon, and nutmeg.

Bring mixture to a simmer, reduce heat, and continue to cook for 5 minutes, stirring regularly while the mixture forms into a syrup.

Peel and core the upper half of each apple and place apples in a shallow baking pan. Pour syrup mixture into the cored center of each apple and any remaining syrup into the bottom of the pan.

Bake, uncovered, for 35 to 40 minutes. Serve warm.

Makes 4 servings
Calories: 188; Protein: .5 gram; Carbohydrates: 44 grams; Fat: 3 grams; Fiber: 3 grams

Apple Crisp

HIGHER FAT   VEGETARIAN   HIGH-FIBER

vegetable oil cooking spray

6 apples, peeled, cored, and sliced

1½ cups rolled oats

½ cup brown sugar

¼ cup all-purpose flour

1 teaspoon cinnamon

½ teaspoon nutmeg

dash salt

4 tablespoons margarine, softened

Preheat oven to 375°F. Spray 8-inch-square baking pan with cooking spray.

Arrange apples evenly in bottom of baking pan.   *(continued)*

Combine oats, brown sugar, flour, cinnamon, nutmeg, and salt in large resealable plastic bag. Add softened margarine. Mix well by massaging outside of bag until mixture is well blended.

Pour oat mixture over sliced apples. Bake 40 to 45 minutes or until topping is lightly browned.

Cool slightly before serving.

Makes 6 servings
Calories: 307; Protein: 4 grams; Carbohydrates: 55 grams; Fat: 9 grams; Fiber: 5 grams

Carrot Raisin Cake

VEGETARIAN

vegetable oil cooking spray

2 cups all-purpose flour

2 cups sugar

1 cup unsweetened applesauce, not chunky

$\frac{1}{2}$ cup vegetable oil

2 eggs

2 teaspoons baking soda

2 teaspoons cinnamon

$\frac{1}{2}$ teaspoon nutmeg

$\frac{1}{2}$ teaspoon salt

3 cups finely grated carrots (about 1 pound)

$\frac{1}{2}$ cup raisins

Icing: (optional)

1 cup confectioners' sugar

1 8-ounce package low-fat cream cheese

1 teaspoon vanilla extract

Preheat oven to 350°F. Spray 9-by-13-inch baking pan with cooking spray.

In large bowl, using an electric mixer, combine flour, sugar, applesauce, oil, eggs, baking soda, cinnamon, nutmeg, and salt. Blend until smooth. Add carrots and raisins. Mix until just combined.

Pour batter into prepared pan. Bake 40 to 45 minutes or until toothpick inserted comes out clean. Cool completely.

If desired, mix icing ingredients and spread over cooled cake. Or you can sprinkle top of cake with 1 tablespoon confectioners' sugar for a finished look.

Makes 24 servings
Calories: 173; Protein: 2 grams; Carbohydrates: 30 grams; Fat: 5 grams; Fiber: .5 gram

RESOURCES AND WEB SITES

Referral Organizations

American Dietetic Association
216 West Jackson Boulevard
Chicago, IL 60604
800/366-1655
www.eatright.org

American Academy of Pediatrics
141 Northwest Point Boulevard
P.O. Box 747
Elk Grove Village, IL 60007
800/433-9016
www.aap.org

The President's Council on
  Physical Fitness and Sports
200 Independence Avenue, SW
Washington, DC 20201
202/690-9000

American College of Sports
  Medicine
c/o Public Information Office
P.O. Box 1440
Indianapolis, Indiana 46206

Anorexia Nervosa and Related
  Eating Disorders, Inc.
P.O. Box 5102
Eugene, OR 97405
541/344-1144
www.anred.com

National Association of Anorexia
  Nervosa and Associated
  Disorders
Box 7
Highland Park, IL 60035
847/831-3438
www.anad.org

The Food Allergy Network
10400 Eaton Place, Suite 107
Fairfax, VA 22030
703/691-3179
800/929-4040
www.foodallergy.org

Allergy and Asthma Network
3554 Chain Bridge Road
  Suite 2000
Fairfax, VA 22030
800/878-4403

American Academy of Allergy,
  Asthma and Immunology
611 East Wells Street
Milwaukee, WI 53202
800/822-ASMA (physician
  referral hotline)
www.aaaai.org

Parents of Asthmatic/
  Allergic Children
1412 Marathon Drive
Fort Collins, CO 80524
303/842-7395

Food and Drug Administration
Office of Consumer Affairs
HFE-88 5600 Fishers Lane
Rockville, MD 20857
800/FDA-4010 (food
  information hotline)
www.fda.gov

Center for Food Safety and
  Applied Nutrition
200 C Street, SW
Washington, DC 20204
www.cfsan.fda.gov

Weight Control Information
  Network
1 Win Way
Bethesda, MD 20892-3665
301/984-7378
800/WIN-8098
www.niddk.nih.gov/health/
  nutrit/win.htm

Vegetarian Resource Group
P.O. Box 1463
Baltimore, MD 21203
410/366-8343
www.vrg.org

Informational Web Sites

Eating Disorders Awareness and
  Prevention Web Site
800/931-2237
www.edap.org
  Offers useful information
when seeking help for eating
disorder treatment.

International Food
  Information Council
www.ific.org
  Collects and disseminates
scientific information on food
safety, nutrition, and health.

Fast Food Finders
www.olen.com/food/
   Helps consumers find nutrient information on fast foods.

Cyber Diet
www.cyberdiet.com/ffq
   Answers questions about healthy lifestyles, and checks calorie content, fat grams, carbohydrates, and more of popular restaurant and fast food fare.

Ask a Dietitian
www.dietitian.com
   Responds to questions via e-mail. Advice on topics such as child nutrition, allergies, weight loss, eating disorders, vegetarianism, exercise, and more.

Vegetarianism
www.planetveggie.com
   Has articles on adopting a vegetarian diet, raising vegetarian kids, and growing organic foods.

Home Food Safety Hotline
800/366-1655
www.homefoodsafety.org
   Offers information, interactive quizzes, glossary of terms, and links to other sites regarding home food safety.

Children's Health
www.kidshealth.org
   Provides latest information for children, teens, and parents on raising healthy children or how to be a healthy child.

Shape Up America
www.shapeup.org
   Provides information on safe weight management, healthy eating, and increased activity and physical fitness.

Calorie Control Council
www.caloriecontrol.org
   Helps in planning low-fat meals and diets, and creating exercise programs.

Nutrition Education
www.navigator.tufts.edu
   Reviews nutrition sites from Tufts University experts. Site for parents, children, and health professionals on nutrition, special diet needs, and more.

Kids CyberClub
www.kidsfood.org
   Interactive site for parents and children makes learning about nutrition both fun and informative.

Girl Power
www.health.org/gpower
   Sponsored by the U.S. Department of Health and Human Services to help encourage and motivate nine- to fourteen-year-old girls make the most of their lives.

Eat 5 A Day for Better Health
www.5aday.com
   Teaches children about good nutrition and 5 A Day fruit and vegetable consumption.

ABOUT THE AUTHORS

Sandra K. Nissenberg, M.S., R.D. is a registered dietitian and nutrition consultant. She spends much of her time working with childhood nutrition issues and has written or cowritten several books in that area including *Quick Meals for Healthy Kids and Busy Parents, I Made It Myself,* and *Brown Bag Success.* Sandy lives in Buffalo Grove, Illinois, with her husband and two children.

Barbara N. Pearl, M.S., R.D. is a registered dietitian and nutrition consultant. She has a private nutrition practice where she counsels children, teens, and adults in all areas of nutrition. Coauthor of *Brown Bag Success,* Barb spends her time lecturing and teaching classes in nutrition at local schools and institutions. Barb lives in Buffalo Grove, Illinois, with her husband and two teenagers.

INDEX

Note: The Index to Recipes begins on page 225.

Index to Recipes